Dear Doctor,

Today's medical practice requires an unprecedented amount of knowledge and ready access to more and more information.

We hope this book will serve as a useful reference source and that you will find it helpful in the course of your busy schedule. It is arranged to provide a myriad of practical details quickly and easily so that your attention can remain focused on the job at hand.

Please accept it with our best wishes.

Very truly yours,

Thomas A. Overmyer

Thomas A. Overmyer
Product Manager
ZANTAC® Tablets
(ranitidine HCl)

Provided as a service to medicine by Glaxo Pharmaceuticals, manufacturers of ZANTAC®.

Health Care Through Discovery and Innovation.

Paul Tucker

6616328

Case Studies in Gastroenterology for the House Officer

Harris R. Clearfield, M.D.

Division of Gastroenterology
Hahnemann University Hospital
Philadelphia, Pennsylvania

Larry M. Borowsky, M.D.

Division of Gastroenterology
Hahnemann University Hospital
Philadelphia, Pennsylvania

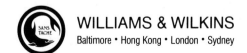

WILLIAMS & WILKINS
Baltimore • Hong Kong • London • Sydney

Editor: Kimberly Kist
Associate Editor: Victoria M. Vaughn
Copy Editor: Emily Ann Donaldson
Illustration Planning: Lorraine Wrzosek
Production: Barbara Felton
Cover Design: Dan Pfisterer

Copyright © 1989
Williams & Wilkins
428 East Preston Street
Baltimore, Maryland 21202, USA

Printed in the United States of America

Library of Congress Cataloging-in-Publication Data

Clearfield, Harris R.
    Case studies in gastroenterology for the house officer.
    Includes index.
    1. Gastrointestinal system—Diseases—Case studies.
I. Borowsky, Larry M. II. Title. [DNLM: 1. Gastroenterology—case studies. WI 100 C623c]
RC808.C54   1989   616.3'309   88-28010
ISBN 0-683-01714-4

89   90   91   92   93
2 3 4 5 6 7 8 9 10

Series Editor's Foreword

The series, Case Studies for the House Officer, has been designed to teach medicine by a case study approach. It is considered a supplement to the parent House Officer Series which provided information in a problem-oriented format. In Case Studies in Gastroenterology for the House Officer, Doctors Clearfield and Borowsky have compiled an impressive series of interesting cases that cover the most common gastroenterology problems. They have added thoughtful "Pearls" and "Pitfalls" and pertinent x-rays, ultrasounds and biopsies as "Clues." The book should be a useful and enjoyable learning experience for students of gastroenterology.

Lawrence P. Levitt, M.D.
Senior Consultant in Neurology
Lehigh Valley Hospital Center
Allentown, Pennsylvania

Clinical Professor of Neurology
Hahnemann University and
Clinical Associate Professor
Temple University School of Medicine
Philadelphia, Pennsylvania

The companion volume to this book is Gastroenterology for the House Officer by David B. Sacher, M.D., and Jerome D. Wayne, M.D.

About the Authors

Harris R. Clearfield, M.D., is a graduate of Franklin and Marshall College and Jefferson Medical College. His medical residency and gastroenterology fellowship were served at the Graduate Hospital of the University of Pennsylvania. He is Professor of Medicine, Director of the Division of Gastroenterology, and Director of the Krancer Center for Inflammatory Bowel Disease Research at Hahnemann University. Dr. Clearfield has twice received the Lindback Foundation Award for distinguished teaching, as well as the Golden Apple Award from the senior class and teaching awards from the junior class.

Larry M. Borowsky, M.D., is a graduate of the University of Pennsylvania and Hahnemann University. He also served his medical residency and gastroenterology fellowship at Hahnemann University, where he is presently Clinical Assistant Professor of Medicine. Dr. Borowsky has been Head of the Endoscopy Unit and currently plays an active role in student and house staff instruction.

Preface

The presentation of a clinical problem combined with an opportunity for reader interaction can be an effective educational tool. Case Studies in Gastroenterology for the House Officer evolved from a series of teaching modules that we have been using for many years. A wide variety of disorders encountered on a gastroenterology service are presented, with the hope that the questions and answers are pertinent to a house officer's interests. The Pearls and Pitfalls sections are designed to highlight important aspects of each case, recognizing that a comprehensive approach is not possible in this format. The Suggested Readings should assist the reader in obtaining additional information. This book is intended to supplement the excellent gastroenterology textbooks available to our house staff and is based on the concept that information directly related to the diagnosis and treatment of a specific patient's problem may be more easily assimilated.

Acknowledgments

We thank our students and house staff, who have shown interest in the concept of teaching modules and stimulated us to proceed with this book. We are also indebted to Jeanne Brigandi for her superb secretarial and administrative assistance. Dr. Steven Teplick from the Department of Radiology and Dr. Simin Dadparvar from the Department of Nuclear Medicine were most helpful in selecting many of the imaging clues. We particularly thank our wives and families for their support and understanding.

Contents

CASE 1: A TEENAGER WITH RECTAL BLEEDING

A 17-year-old female high school student presented with the complaint of bright red rectal bleeding associated with several soft or loose stools per day and lower abdominal discomfort of 2 weeks duration. There was no history of antibiotic use, fever or joint discomfort. There was no unusual travel history. Physical examination showed normal vital signs and no abnormality of the chest or heart. There was slight tenderness in the left lower quadrant. A digital rectal examination revealed red blood on the examining finger.

BARIUM ENEMA CLUE

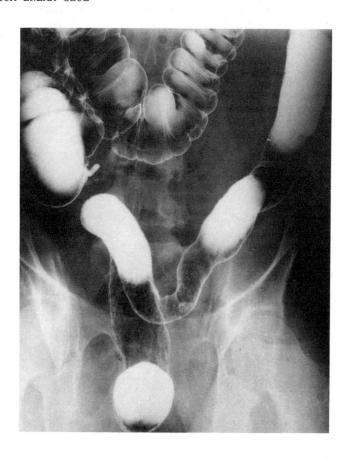

QUESTIONS (Please read the corresponding answer before proceeding to the next question.)

1. What are the most likely possibilities?

2. What studies are most important at this time?

3. Can bacterial and parasitic infections produce these sigmoidoscopy findings?

4. Should rectal steroids be started?

5. Should antibiotics be given?

6. Should you prescribe sulfasalazine?

7. Should you order a barium enema examination?

ANSWERS

1. Amebiasis (even without a travel history), ulcerative colitis and infectious diarrheas such as Shigella, Salmonella and campylobacter.

2. A complete blood count (CBC) and stool examination for culture, sensitivity, ova, and parasites should be obtained. A sigmoidoscopy should also be performed (in this case it showed petechial hemorrhages, mild exudate, edema and hyperemia without ulcerations).

3. The sigmoidoscopic findings in Shigella, Salmonella, campylobacter and amebiasis may be normal or could closely resemble ulcerative colitis.

4. Not when the possibility of bacterial or parasitic infection exists.

5. Antibiotics should be withheld since the diagnosis has not been established. Salmonella gastroenteritis should not be treated with antibiotics since a carrier state may result. Salmonella bacteremia, however, should be treated with ampicillin. Moderate or severe cases of shigellosis are usually treated with trimethoprim/sulfamethoxazole. Campylobacter enterocolitis often subsides spontaneously but does respond to erythromycin.

6. If ulcerative colitis is suspected, sulfasalazine can be started before the results of the stool examinations are available, as was done in this case. The stool examinations were negative and the patient gradually improved on 8 weeks of sulfasalazine therapy, confirming the impression of ulcerative colitis. Hydrocortisone enemas have also been useful for rectosigmoid involvement. More recently, 5-aminosalicylic acid enemas have been found to be equally effective without the corticosteroid side effects.

7. There is no urgency for a barium enema. The barium will interfere with stool examination for parasites and the laxative preparation will be difficult to tolerate. If stool examinations are negative (as they were in this patient) the response to therapy can be monitored with flexible sigmoidoscopy. A barium enema can be obtained later in the course of therapy, as was done in this case, to serve as a baseline study. It showed ulcerations in the rectum, sigmoid colon and distal

descending colon as well as some loss of distensibility (see Clue).

PEARLS

1. The ulcerations of Crohn's disease are more severe than those of ulcerative colitis. The rectal inflammation is confluent in ulcerative colitis and tends to be patchy in Crohn's disease (which can involve the rectum).

2. Sigmoidoscopic examinations should be performed without a cleansing enema in patients with suspected inflammatory bowel disease, since the enema itself often produces hyperemia and mucus secretion.

3. Do not forget the possibility of anal gonorrhea, a disorder that largely involves the crypts and is accompanied by bleeding and purulent exudate. It does not, however, extend significantly into the rectal ampulla, as described in this patient.

4. The history of loose stools suggests that the inflammatory process is not limited to the rectum (ulcerative proctitis) since formed stools would be expected with very distal disease.

5. When initiating sulfasalazine therapy for ulcerative colitis, one should begin with small doses, such as 0.5 g 3 times daily for several days and increase gradually to 1.0 g 4 times daily. Watch for nausea, indigestion and headache secondary to the sulfa component.

PITFALLS

1. Do not initiate antidiarrheal therapy for known or suspected diarrhea due to campylobacter, Salmonella, Shigella or Yersinia. Diphenoxylate slows colonic transit and may cause overgrowth of the pathogens.

2. Although pseudomembranes are the hallmark of Clostridium difficile colitis, some patients present with sigmoidoscopic findings indistinguishable from ulcerative colitis.

3. Sulfasalazine should be the first-line drug for mild to moderately severe ulcerative colitis. Do not start steroids immediately since it may be difficult to

reduce or stop therapy because of "rebound" symptoms. Steroids, however, should be used as initial therapy for severe ulcerative colitis.

4. There is no need to severely restrict the diet of patients with rectosigmoid ulcerative colitis. The elimination of roughage can be useful if there is a tendency to diarrhea.

SUGGESTED READINGS

Booth IW, Harries JT: Inflammatory bowel disease in childhood. Gut 25:188, 1984.
Campieri M, Gionchetti P, Belluzzi A, et al: Efficacy of 5-aminosalicylic enema versus hydrocortisone enemas in ulcerative colitis. Dig Dis Sci 32:675, 1987.
Glickman RM: Inflammatory bowel disease. In Braunwald E, et al (eds): Harrison's Principles of Internal Medicine, ed. 11. New York, McGraw-Hill, 1987, pp 1277-1290.
Lebedeff DA, Hochman EB: Rectal gonorrhea in men: Diagnosis and treatment. Ann Int Med 92:463, 1980.
Lennard-Jones JE: Toward optimal use of corticosteroids in ulcerative colitis and Crohn's disease. Gut 24:177, 1983.
Peppercorn MA: Sulfasalazine. Ann Int Med 3:377, 1984.
Peppercorn MA: Current status of drug therapy for inflammatory bowel disease. Compr Ther 11:14, 1985.

CASE 2: A SMOKER WITH RECURRENT UPPER ABDOMINAL PAIN

A 43-year-old accountant had experienced intermittent
episodes of abdominal pain during the previous 10 years and
treated himself with frequent antacids. He was comfortable
for several years until 3 months prior to his visit when he
noted the onset of recurrent episodes of more severe upper
abdominal discomfort which were usually relieved by eating
and, more recently, awakened him from sleep. The pain was
not well-localized, lasted 15 to 30 minutes, and did not
radiate to the back or chest. He took no analgesic
medications, was a social drinker and smoked 1 package of
cigarettes per day. There is no family history of peptic
ulcer. Physical examination showed no abnormality of the
chest or heart. The abdomen was soft, the liver and spleen
were not enlarged and no tenderness could be elicited. A
rectal examination showed brown stool which was negative
for occult blood.

BARIUM UPPER GI CLUE

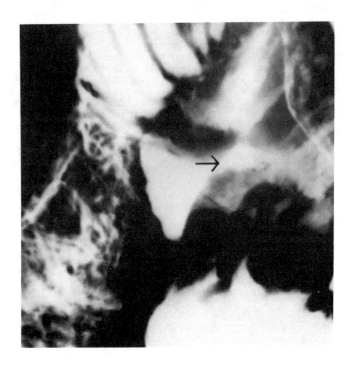

QUESTIONS (Please read the corresponding answer before proceeding to the next question.)

1. What diagnoses would you consider?

2. Should you start therapy based on the history and physical examination, obtain an upper GI x-ray or perform an upper gastrointestinal endoscopy?

3. Would you treat with antacids, H2-receptor antagonists, or sucralfate?

4. What role does smoking play in the genesis and healing rate of duodenal ulcer disease?

5. Should this patient be placed on maintenance therapy, once healing has occurred, to prevent recurrent ulcer disease?

ANSWERS

1. Recurrent epigastric pain relieved by food and awakening the patient from sleep should suggest peptic ulcer disease. Pancreatitis is always a possibility when recurrent upper abdominal pain is described. Although nonulcer dyspepsia can mimic ulcer disease, the nocturnal pain makes a functional etiology less likely.

2. A patient who describes the recent onset of pain which is suggestive of peptic ulcer disease may be empirically treated with the understanding that symptoms should respond rapidly to appropriate therapy. Indeed, failure to respond in several days should suggest that the diagnosis is incorrect or that the ulcer disease is complicated. This patient has had recurrent and undiagnosed discomfort and should be studied by either upper gastrointestinal endoscopy or barium meal examination. The latter was obtained in this patient and showed evidence of an acute ulcer in a deformed duodenal bulb (see Clue).

3. Seven-dose antacid therapy (1 and 3 hours after meals and at bedtime), H2-receptor antagonists (cimetidine, famotidine or ranitidine), and sucralfate are equally effective, achieving a duodenal ulcer healing rate of approximately 90% in 8 weeks. Outpatient compliance is poor for antacids; therefore, sucralfate or H2-receptor antagonists should be considered for this patient.

4. Cigarette smoking delays the healing of duodenal ulcers and promotes recurrences. One explanation is that cigarettes inhibit pancreatic secretion of bicarbonate, thus diminishing the buffering capacity of the duodenal fluids, resulting in a lower duodenal pH.

5. Duodenal ulcer disease should be viewed as a chronic disorder with a high rate of recurrence (up to 75% in 1 year). Risk factors such as smoking, older age group and family history of duodenal ulcer increase the probability of recurrence. The patient should be strongly encouraged to stop smoking. Although maintenance therapy should not be started after the 1st ulcer heals, recurrent disease should prompt long-term treatment with an H2-receptor antagonist. A serum gastrin should be obtained to exclude the Zollinger-Ellison syndrome.

PEARLS

1. Nocturnal ulcer pain must be treated with H2-receptor antagonists rather than antacids since a prolonged acid suppression effect is required.

2. Although duodenal ulcer pain usually subsides rapidly with effective therapy, healing may be much slower. Therapy should be continued for 6 to 8 weeks.

3. It is difficult to distinguish between gastric and duodenal ulcer disease on the basis of the history and physical examination. Prepyloric and duodenal ulcers are only a few centimeters apart and epigastric tenderness is not a specific predictor for peptic ulcer. A consideration of "peptic disease" is sufficient, since x-ray or endoscopy can localize the pathology.

4. Although complete cessation of smoking is desirable for the treatment of peptic ulcer, the effects appear to be dose related, so that a decrease to 10 cigarettes per day or less would be helpful.

5. Back pain in a patient with active peptic disease should suggest the possibility of pancreatitis resulting from posterior ulcer penetration to the pancreas. The amylase is normal in approximately 50% of such cases so that an elevation should not be regarded as necessary for the diagnosis.

PITFALLS

1. Typical ulcer symptoms in the absence of demonstrable peptic disease are referred to as nonulcer dyspepsia. Many such patients are treated chronically and inappropriately with H2-receptor antagonists.

2. Cimetidine's effect on cytochrome P-450, one of the hepatic enzymes responsible for drug metabolism, results in higher blood levels of many therapeutic agents. Ranitidine would be a safer choice when H2-receptor antagonist therapy is indicated for patients receiving other drugs with a narrow therapeutic range.

3. Although duodenal ulcers which have been treated for an adequate period of time do not require endoscopic or radiographic evidence of healing, gastric ulcers should

be re-endoscoped after 8 weeks of therapy to confirm
healing and for rebiopsy to exclude the possibility of
malignancy.

SUGGESTED READINGS

Brooks FP: The pathophysiology of peptic ulcer disease.
    Dig Dis Sci 30 (Nov 1985 Supplement):15S, 1985.
Freston JW: H2-receptor antagonists and duodenal ulcer
    recurrence: Analysis of efficacy and commentary on
    safety, costs, and patient selection. Am J
    Gastroenterol 82:1242, 1987.
McGuigan JE: Peptic Ulcer. In Braunwald E, et al (eds):
    Harrison's Principles of Internal Medicine, ed. 11.
    New York, McGraw-Hill, 1987, pp 1239-1253.
Priebe WM, DaCosta LR, Beck IT: Is epigastric tenderness a
    sign of peptic ulcer disease? Gastroenterology
    82:16, 1982.
Sax MJ: Clinically important adverse effects and drug
    interactions with H2-receptor antagonists.
    Pharmacotherapy 7:110S, 1987.
Siepler JK, Mahakian K, Trudeau WT: Current concepts in
    clinical therapeutics: Peptic ulcer disease. Clin
    Pharmacol 5:128, 1986.
Sontag S, Graham DY, Belsito A, et al: Cimetidine,
    cigarette smoking, and recurrence of duodenal ulcer.
    N Engl J Med 311:689, 1984.
Walt R, Logan R, Katachinski B, et al: Rising frequency of
    ulcer perforation in elderly people in the United
    Kingdom. Lancet 1:489, 1986.

CASE 3: A VERY SOCIAL DRINKER WITH ABDOMINAL PAIN AND
VOMITING

A 32-year-old construction worker is admitted to the
hospital because of severe upper abdominal pain radiating
to the back, and recurrent vomiting. He has been admitted
to other hospitals several times in the past year for
similar complaints and was told he had pancreatitis. He
drinks approximately 1 pint of whiskey daily on weekends
and several drinks nightly on weekdays, but his alcohol
intake had been greater in the past. He underwent a
cholecystectomy at age 24 for gallstones. Physical
examination showed his blood pressure 150/90, pulse 92, and
temperature 99.6 F. No spider nevi were present. Bowel
sounds were hypoactive and there was considerable
tenderness in the upper abdomen. The liver measured 12 cm
in the midclavicular line and the spleen was not enlarged.
A digital rectal examination was negative.

The white blood count was 11,200 with 80 segs, 12 lymphs,
2 bands, and 6 monos. The amylase was 750 units (normal to
100 units), lipase was 5.6 units (normal to 1.0 units),
bilirubin 2.5 mg%, alkaline phosphatase was 80 units
(normal to 80 units), serum glutamic oxaloacetic
transaminase (SGOT, AST) was 150 units and serum glutamic
pyruvic transaminase (SGPT, ALT) was 60 units.

PANCREATIC ULTRASOUND CLUE

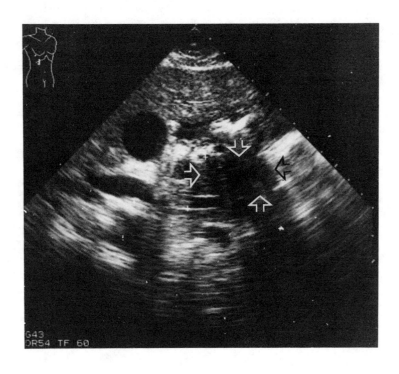

QUESTIONS (Please read the corresponding answer before proceeding to the next question.)

1. Do the biochemical studies support a diagnosis of pancreatitis?

2. What findings on an obstruction series would suggest pancreatitis?

3. Should a nasogastric tube be inserted?

4. What could explain the frequency of the recurrent attacks of pain?

5. What biochemical studies would suggest that this is necrotizing rather than edematous pancreatitis?

6. What probably caused the bilirubin elevation?

ANSWERS

1. The elevation of both amylase and lipase are sufficient
    to establish a diagnosis of pancreatitis. The serum
    lipase, which rises somewhat later than the serum
    amylase in the course of pancreatitis, is a less
    sensitive but more specific test. An ultrasound study
    of the pancreas in this patient showed an edematous
    enlargement of the pancreatic head (see Clue).

2. The presence of pancreatic calcifications, gallstones,
    a left pleural effusion, colon cut-off sign (air in the
    transverse colon which is not seen beyond the mid or
    distal portion, presumably secondary to localized
    colonic ileus) and sentinel loop (localized ileus of
    small bowel, often the duodenal loop).

3. A nasogastric tube is required when ileus and/or
    vomiting are present. In the absence of these
    complications, there is no benefit to nasogastric
    suction. Nasogastric aspiration was used in this
    patient.

4. Recurrence of pancreatitis or a persistently elevated
    serum amylase should suggest the possibility of
    pancreatic pseudocyst (the ultrasound showed no
    evidence of pseudocyst). Continued alcohol intake is
    another possibility. The previous cholecystectomy
    requires consideration of residual common bile duct
    stones (the ultrasound showed no ductal dilation).

5. The acute onset of diabetes, hypocalcemia or
    methemalbuminemia (produces brown serum when very high)
    are strongly suggestive of necrotizing pancreatitis.
    Leukocytosis and jaundice could also suggest a severe
    inflammatory process.

6. The jaundice could be secondary to compression of the
    distal common bile duct by the swollen pancreatic head.
    The SGOT elevation, which is more than twice that of
    the SGPT, also suggests alcoholic hepatitis. A liver
    biopsy confirmed the latter diagnosis.

PEARLS

1. Although the serum amylase may be increased for many
    reasons (vomiting, morphine, intestinal obstruction and

azotemia), elevations of 5 or more times the upper
limit of normal are usually due to pancreatitis.

2. Although acute pancreatitis can cause compression of
the common bile duct, a very high bilirubin resulting
from complete ductal occlusion is uncommon.

3. Acute pancreatitis without any apparent explanation
(idiopathic pancreatitis) is associated with a
mortality rate as high as 20%. Continue to suspect
gallstones in women with unexplained pancreatitis and
negative ultrasound studies. An oral cholecystogram
may prove useful. An endoscopic retrograde
cholangiopancreatogram (ERCP) may demonstrate a
congenital pancreatic ductal anomaly, pancreas divisum.

4. The Grey Turner's sign (bilateral ecchymosis of the
flanks which may extend to the groin) is highly
suggestive of hemorrhagic pancreatitis but has been
described with a ruptured aortic aneurysm.

PITFALLS

1. Morphine increases the tone of the sphincter of Oddi,
thus raising intraductal pressure and perhaps
exacerbating the inflammatory process, and should not
be given to patients with pancreatitis.
Anticholinergics (once used in an attempt to relax the
sphincter) are contraindicated because of their
propensity to induce ileus.

2. Patients with necrotizing pancreatitis may lose
sufficient protein and fluid into the abdomen and other
tissues to induce hypotension. Colloid should be given
to maintain the circulating blood volume.

3. Refeeding too soon after the pain begins to improve is
a cause for relapse. Consider total parenteral
nutrition if the pancreatitis is moderate or severe.

4. Patients with recurrent alcoholic pancreatitis are
easily addicted to narcotics.

5. Once patients are clinically recovered and tolerate
feedings without difficulty, the hospitalization need
not be delayed because of continued amylase elevation.
Some patients maintain such elevations for variable
periods of time without relationship to their symptoms.

SUGGESTED READINGS

Beger HG, Bittner R, Block S, et al: Bacterial
    contamination of pancreatic necrosis. A prospective
    clinical study. Gastroenterology 91:433, 1986.
Blamey SL, Imrie CW, O'Neill J, et al: Prognostic factors
    in acute pancreatitis. Gut 25:1340, 1984.
Clark LR, Jaffe MH, Choyke PL, et al: Pancreatic imaging.
    Radiologic Clin North Am 23:489, 1985.
Corfield AP, Cooper MJ, Williamson RCN: Acute
    pancreatitis: A lethal disease of increasing
    incidence. Gut 26:724, 1985.
Geokas MC, Baltaxe HA, Banks PA, et al: Acute
    pancreatitis. Ann Int Med 103:86, 1985.
Gerzof SG, Banks PA, Robbins AH, et al: Early diagnosis of
    pancreatic infection by computed tomography-guided
    aspiration. Gastroenterology 93:1315, 1987.
Mayer AD, McMahon MJ, Corfield AP, et al: Controlled
    clinical trial of peritoneal lavage for the treatment
    of severe acute pancreatitis. N Engl J Med
    312:399, 1985.
Moosa AR: Diagnostic tests and procedures in acute
    pancreatitis. N Engl J Med 311:639, 1984.

CASE 4:   JAUNDICE IN A HYPERTENSIVE HOMOSEXUAL PATIENT

A 37-year-old male presents with a 10-day history of
anorexia, fatigue, malaise, low grade fever, dark urine and
upper abdominal discomfort. There is no history of
jaundice, intravenous drug use or blood transfusions. He
is homosexual. Alcohol intake consists of several mixed
drinks nightly and wine with dinner. Hypertension was
detected 2 years ago and he has been taking
hydrochlorothiazide and alpha-methyldopa.

Physical examination includes: temperature of 99.6F, blood
pressure 150/80. He is icteric. No spider nevi are
detected. The liver measures 12 cm in the midclavicular
line and is moderately tender. The spleen is not palpable.

Initial laboratory data: total bilirubin = 6.8 mg%;
alkaline phosphatase = 240 units (normal to 85 units); AST
(SGOT) = 980 units (normal to 40 units); ALT (SGPT) = 1200
units (normal to 40 units). The white blood count is 5,600
with a normal differential count.

CLUE

Closer questioning reveals that the patient had experienced several days of joint stiffness, primarily in the fingers, prior to his presenting symptoms.

QUESTIONS (Please read the corresponding answer before proceeding to the next question.)

1. What information do you derive from the initial laboratory studies?

2. What are the diagnostic possibilities?

3. What additional studies would you obtain?

4. If this patient was subsequently found to have AIDS, how might this influence your differential diagnosis?

5. What is the delta virus?

6. Your senior medical student inadvertently sustained a needle stick from a syringe used to draw blood from this patient. What would you advise him to do?

ANSWERS

1. The alkaline phosphatase is over twice the top normal
    value, indicating a significant degree of cholestasis.
    (Although the alkaline phosphatase elevation could be
    secondary to bone disease, the associated biochemical
    evidence of liver injury makes this an unlikely
    consideration). The SGOT and SGPT are both well over
    10 times the top normal value, thus reflecting a major
    degree of liver injury. No specific diagnosis can be
    made from "liver function tests" (more descriptively
    called "liver injury tests") other than to indicate
    whether the process is cholestatic or inflammatory. In
    this case, there is evidence for both mechanisms.

2. a. Acute drug-induced hepatitis secondary to alpha-
    methyldopa.
    b. Acute viral hepatitis (A, B or non-A, non-B)
    c. Biliary tract obstruction with ascending
    cholangitis. Tenderness, jaundice, obstructive and
    inflammatory biochemical abnormalities are compatible
    with this diagnosis, but the normal white blood count
    and low grade fever makes this possibility less likely.

3. Initial serologic studies were as follows:
    a. IgM antibody to hepatitis A virus (which was
    negative).
    b. HBsAg (which was positive), anti-HBs (negative),
    and IgM anti-HBc (positive).
    c. A prothrombin time (normal in this case) should be
    performed in all cases of acute hepatitis since, if
    prolonged, it could reflect severe liver damage.
    d. These studies reflect an acute hepatitis B. Had
    they been negative, an ultrasound of the biliary tract
    would have been performed.

4. Liver biopsies are abnormal in approximately 85% of
    AIDS patients. Evidence of HBV exposure (antigens or
    antibodies) are found in almost 90% of such patients,
    but the frequency of chronic active hepatitis appears
    to be no greater than that found in immunocompetent
    adults. Specific AIDS-related disease is found in
    approximately 40% of patients, with mycobacterium
    avium-intracellulare the most frequent pathogen seen,
    but Kaposi's sarcoma is among the most common
    postmortem hepatic findings. Cytomegalovirus (CMV)
    and hepatic mycoses have been less frequently observed.
    Liver biopsies are not indicated for the evaluation of
    minor liver function abnormalities since the findings

are frequently nonspecific or fail to effect a change in therapy.

5. The hepatitis delta virus (HDV) is composed of an RNA genome and delta antigen, with an outer coat of HBsAg obtained from HBV. The obligatory association of HDV with HBV occurs during simultaneous infection with both viruses or HDV infection superimposed on an HBsAg carrier. Although the clinical picture with acute coinfection is similar to that for HBV alone, superinfection with HDV is one of the considerations for an acute exacerbation of a chronic HBV hepatitis. Such patients are more likely to proceed to chronic active hepatitis and cirrhosis.

6. If the student has been immunized, he should be tested for anti-HBs. If an inadequate antibody is found, 1 dose (0.06 ml/kg) of HBIG (hepatitis B immune globulin) should be given immediately, as well as a hepatitis B vaccine booster dose. If he has not been immunized, he should be given 1 dose of HBIG immediately and a hepatitis B vaccine series should be initiated. Immunized individuals at high risk for contacting hepatitis B should have their anti-HBs levels evaluated yearly. A recent study showed that 38% of hospital workers had diminished antibody levels 3 years after vaccination. If an inadequate antibody response is found following the 1st series of hepatitis B vaccine, revaccination will be successful in approximately 50%. Interval booster doses may be required for some individuals.

PEARLS

1. It may be important to inquire as to cocaine use in patients with unexplained hepatitis since cocaine toxicity has now been reported to result in hepatic as well as cardiac, renal, intestinal and cerebral damage. Cocaine-induced hepatotoxicity produces periportal necrosis.

2. An individual who has sustained a needle stick from a patient with known non-A, non-B hepatitis should be given immune globulin at a dose of 0.06 ml/kg as soon as possible after the exposure even though the value of this passive immunization is uncertain. It is theorized that there may be sufficient antibody in the preparation to provide immunization against the unknown agent responsible for the hepatitis.

3. The availability of a more sensitive radioimmunoassay has demonstrated a higher percentage of concurrent HBsAg and anti-HBs in acute and chronic hepatitis B disease. The "serologic window" in acute hepatitis B (the time between the disappearance of the surface antigen and the appearance of the surface antibody) is probably shorter than previously recognized. Hepatitis B e (HBeAg) antigen occurs more frequently in patients with concurrent markers than in those with HBsAg alone, indicating a higher likelihood of active viral replication. The concurrence may be constant or intermittent and is more common in patients with chronic active hepatitis than in those with chronic persistent hepatitis or asymptomatic carriers.

4. Some patients with chronic HBsAg and HBeAg in the serum, particularly immunosuppressed individuals, have little evidence of chronic liver disease. This appears to represent a deficient immunologic response to viral replication and supports the contention that hepatitis is not the result of the virus but represents the immunologic response to viral replication.

PITFALLS

1. The conversion of HBeAg to anti-HBe in patients with chronic hepatitis B occurs with a frequency of approximately 13% per year and is thought to represent evidence of subsiding inflammation. A reactivation rate, however, of approximately 30% within 18 months of loss of HBeAg has been reported, although often associated with mild biochemical evidence of disease activity. Such patients may fail to redevelop anti-HBe.

2. Serum biochemical "liver function tests" are often used to distinguish between healthy HBV carriers and those with HBV liver disease. The height of ALT and AST elevation does not always correlate with the degree of liver damage and some patients with chronic type B hepatitis have periods when these enzymes are near normal. To further complicate the distinction, some patients with chronic persistent type B hepatitis may later be found to have chronic active hepatitis. A liver biopsy is required if the distinction is to be made with greater confidence.

3. The pain of acute viral (or alcoholic) hepatitis may be sufficiently severe, due to the stretching of Glisson's capsule, to mimic acute cholecystitis.

4. The clay-colored stools experienced by patients with acute viral hepatitis may be erroneously ascribed to extrahepatic bile duct obstruction. The intrahepatic inflammation and edema resulting from viral hepatitis may exert sufficient pressure to cause transient compression of the bile canaliculi, thus inhibiting bile flow.

SUGGESTED READINGS

Fagan EA, Williams R: Serological responses to HBV infection. Gut 27:858, 1986.
Hoofnagle JH, Shafritz DA, Popper H: Chronic type B hepatitis and the "healthy" HBsAg carrier state. Hepatology 7:758, 1987.
Horowitz MM, Ershler WB, McKinney WP, et al: Duration of immunity after hepatitis B vaccination: Efficacy of low-dose booster vaccine. Ann Int Med 108:185, 1988.
Lok ASF, Lai CL, Wu PC, et al: Spontaneous hepatitis B e antigen to antibody seroconversion and reversion in Chinese patients with chronic hepatitis B virus infection. Gastroenterology 92:1839, 1987.
Perino LE, Warren GH, Levine JS: Cocaine-induced hepatotoxicity in humans. Gastroenterology 93:176, 1987.
Schiff E: Immunoprophylaxis of viral hepatitis: A practical guide. Am J Gastroenterol 82:287, 1987.
Schneiderman DJ, Arenson DM, Cello JP, et al: Hepatic disease in patients with the acquired immune deficiency syndrome (AIDS). Hepatology 7:925, 1987.
Shiels MK, Taswell HF, Czaja AJ, et al: Frequency and significance of concurrent hepatitis B surface antigen and antibody in acute and chronic hepatitis B. Gastroenterology 93:675, 1987.

CASE 5: DYSPHAGIA: MOTILITY, INFLAMMATORY OR NEOPLASTIC?

A 47-year-old woman presents with the complaint of
increasing low substernal dysphagia for the past 14 months.
The symptom had been occasional at the onset, but has been
almost daily during the preceding several months and occurs
with both liquids and solids. There is no heartburn or
chest discomfort. Regurgitation has occurred during sleep.
She has lost approximately 10 pounds in the last 6 months.
An upper GI barium x-ray was performed 1 year ago and she
was told that it was normal. Her symptoms have been
ascribed to "tension." The physical examination was
unremarkable.

BARIUM UPPER GI CLUE

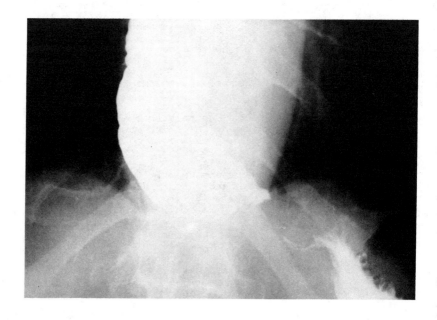

QUESTIONS (Please read the corresponding answer before proceeding to the next question.)

1. What physical findings might be clues to the diagnosis of esophageal complaints?

2. What is your differential diagnosis?

3. If this is achalasia, what would you expect an upper GI barium x-ray to show?

4. Achalasia is now suspected.   What would you expect an upper GI endoscopy to show?

5. What would you expect the esophageal motility study to show if this is achalasia?

6. What pharmacologic agents could be tried?

7. What therapy would you advise now?

8. What symptoms may develop after treatment of achalasia?

ANSWERS

1. Evidence of pharyngeal candidiasis could be a helpful
    clue. The skin changes of scleroderma can be a useful
    finding, particularly if Raynaud's phenomenon and
    telangiectasia are present, thus raising the
    possibility of the CREST syndrome (calcinosis,
    Raynaud's phenomenon, esophageal dysmotility,
    scleroderma and telangiectasia). Evidence of anemia
    and "spooned" nails should suggest the Plummer-Vinson
    syndrome, which is associated with a web in the
    cervical esophagus, usually on the anterior wall.

2. a. Achalasia because of the long history, the absence
    of heartburn and her age, which makes carcinoma less
    likely.
    b. Also consider a lower esophageal ring, scleroderma,
    reflux esophagitis (without heartburn) and esophageal
    or gastric carcinoma.

3. The upper GI barium x-ray in this case showed a smooth,
    narrowed terminal esophagus with a tubular dilatation
    of the esophageal body. The barium emptied slowly in
    the erect position and not at all when she was
    recumbent.

4. The upper GI endoscopy was performed to determine if
    there was an inflammatory aspect to the disorder
    (superimposed moniliasis can result in odynophagia) and
    to rule out the possibility of malignancy. In this
    instance the body of the esophagus was normal. The
    instrument passed through the narrowed terminal
    esophagus with gentle pressure and entered the stomach
    easily. There was no evidence of mucosal disease.

5. The esophageal motility examination was performed to
    provide additional information about the motility of
    the body and lower esophageal sphincter (LES). There
    was no observable primary peristalsis (a swallowing-
    initiated peristaltic contraction which begins in the
    proximal esophagus and descends to the stomach). The
    resting pressure in the LES was 40 mm Hg (normal is
    10-20 mm Hg). The pressure in the LES should relax to
    approximately zero when swallowing occurs so that the
    bolus can enter the stomach, but the pressure in this
    patient only relaxed to 25 mm Hg with swallowing.
    These motility findings are compatible with achalasia.

6. Sublingual isosorbide dinitrate and calcium channel inhibitors, such as verapamil and nifedipine, have been useful in reducing LES pressure in achalasia, but the effects are often transient. A trial of therapy in this patient was ineffective.

7. Pneumatic dilatation of the esophagus is preferable to surgery. The forceful stretching of the LES ruptures the circular muscle fibers and achieves satisfactory results in approximately 50% of patients. If this is unsuccessful, a 2nd dilatation should be attempted. Pneumatic dilatation provided complete relief of symptoms in this patient. A Heller-type myotomy (a longitudinal incision of the LES through the muscle fibers down to the mucosa) should be performed if pneumatic dilatation is unsuccessful.

8. Pneumatic dilatation and myotomy both widen the LES, thus permitting gastroesophageal reflux. Some surgeons advocate the combination of a fundoplication with the myotomy.

PEARLS

1. A short history of symptoms prior to the development of significant dysphagia should raise the possibility of malignancy. Carcinomas at the cardioesophageal junction may infiltrate submucosally and produce radiographic and manometric findings compatible with achalasia. This has been referred to as pseudoachalasia.

2. Esophageal strictures usually result initially in dysphagia for solids and gradually lead to difficulty with liquids as the degree of narrowing increases. The early dysphagia in achalasia is usually for both solids and liquids, since the high LES pressure prevents passage of all esophageal contents.

3. Esophageal peristalsis is absent in scleroderma and achalasia, but the LES pressure is low in scleroderma and elevated in achalasia. Gastroesophageal reflux is a problem for many patients with scleroderma and should be managed with chronic H2-receptor antagonist therapy.

4. Patients with untreated achalasia of long duration may occasionally be diagnosed by chest x-ray because of the markedly dilated esophagus which can contain an air-fluid level.

5. Regurgitated food in achalasia does not taste sour
    since it is esophageal rather than gastric in origin.

PITFALLS

1. Even though patients may have radiographic and
    manometric evidence of achalasia, endoscopy should be
    performed to rule out superimposed moniliasis and
    malignancy.

2. Do not forget that achalasia and gastroesophageal
    reflux disease can lead to nocturnal coughing and
    asthmatic episodes resulting from aspiration or reflux
    which stimulates reflux bronchospasm. Severe
    laryngitis and lung abscess may also occur.

3. Although carcinoma may mimic achalasia, there appears
    to be an increased incidence of carcinoma in patients
    with chronic, untreated achalasia, perhaps secondary to
    the prolonged contact of food carcinogens with the
    esophageal mucosa.

4. Chest pain may be an early symptom in some patients and
    could be confused with cardiac disease. This entity
    has been referred to as "vigorous achalasia," but
    probably represents a variant of esophageal spasm in
    combination with achalasia. The pain usually subsides
    as the esophagus dilates.

SUGGESTED READINGS

Donahue PE, Samelson S, Schlesinger PK, et al: Achalasia
    of the esophagus. Treatment controversies and the
    method of choice. Ann Surg 203:505, 1986.
Fellows IW, Ogilvie A L, Atkinson M: Pneumatic dilatation
    in achalasia. Gut 24:1020, 1983.
Gelfond M, Rozen P, Gilat T: Isosorbide dinitrate and
    nifedipine treatment of achalasia: A clinical,
    manometric and radionuclide evaluation.
    Gastroenterology 83:963, 1982.
Kahrilas PJ, Kishk SM, Helm JF: Comparison of
    pseudoachalasia and achalasia. Am J Med 82:439, 1987.

CASE 6:   RECURRENT DUODENAL ULCER AND DIARRHEA

A 43-year-old laborer was diagnosed by upper GI barium
x-ray as having duodenal ulcer disease 2 years ago.   He was
placed on H2-receptor antagonist therapy and became
asymptomatic.   Recurrent symptoms 9 months later prompted
an upper GI endoscopy which showed evidence of another
active duodenal ulcer.   He was placed back on H2-receptor
antagonist therapy for 8 weeks and he was persuaded to stop
smoking.   Symptoms again subsided and he did well until 3
weeks prior to admission when he developed more severe
episodes of upper abdominal pain and mild diarrhea.   There
was no history of alcohol or analgesic use.   Physical
examination in the emergency room showed epigastric
tenderness without evidence of peritonitis.   The CBC,
amylase, and obstruction series were unremarkable.   Upper
GI endoscopy showed antral gastritis, marked duodenitis and
a deeply penetrating duodenal ulcer.

BARIUM UPPER GI CLUE

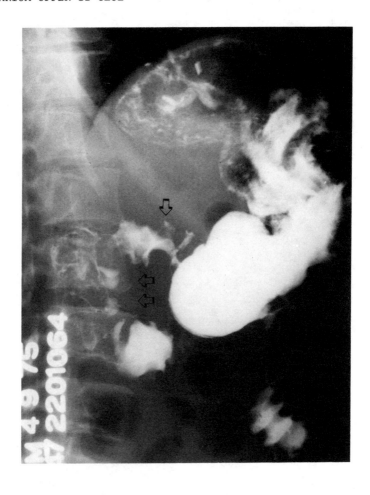

QUESTIONS (Please read the corresponding answer before proceeding to the next question.)

1. What study would be most important at this time?

2. How could you determine the implications of the elevated serum gastrin level?

3. What other disorders would you consider?

4. How can you explain this patient's diarrhea?

5. What studies would you order to anatomically localize a possible tumor?

6. What therapy would you proceed with?

ANSWERS

1. The history of recurrent duodenal ulcer disease
requires a serum gastrin determination. In view of the
variability of the gastrin levels in Zollinger-Ellison
(Z-E) syndrome, a serum gastrin should be performed
daily for several days. The highest serum gastrin in
this patient was 250 pg/ml (normal 20-100 pg/ml). A
basal acid output may also be useful, since values over
15 mEq/hour are strongly suggestive of Z-E syndrome. A
small percentage of duodenal ulcer patients may also
have elevated basal acid outputs, but the maximal acid
output appears to add little to the specificity of
gastric analysis in this disorder. The basal acid
output in this patient was 21 mEq/liter. Other causes
for an elevated basal acid output include retained
gastric antrum, gastric outlet obstruction, renal
failure, short bowel syndrome and antral G cell
hyperplasia.

2. A secretin provocative test should be performed to
confirm the presence of the Z-E syndrome. H2-receptor
antagonist therapy should be stopped prior to the
examination. Patients with duodenal ulcer disease show
little change in their serum gastrin levels after a
bolus of intravenous secretin-Kabi (2 units/kg body
weight), while Z-E patients show a rise of at least
200 pg/ml over basal levels. The secretin provocative
test in this patient showed a rise from the basal value
of 215 pg/ml to 635 pg/ml. An infusion of intravenous
calcium will also stimulate a gastrin increase in Z-E
patients, but the procedure offers no advantages over
the secretin provocative test.

3. The type 1 multiple endocrine neoplasia syndrome
(MEN-1) is found in 15-26% of patients with Z-E
syndrome. Hypercalcemia secondary to
hyperparathyroidism is the most common MEN-1 associated
disorder, with functioning islet cell adenomas of the
pancreas the 2nd most common abnormality. The serum
calcium and phosphate were normal in this patient and
there was no family history to suggest a genetic
disorder.

4. Diarrhea may be a prominent symptom in patients with
severe and chronic Z-E syndrome, but even patients with
mild ulcer disease may experience some diarrhea. The
marked acid output may produce a chemical duodenal
jejunitis. This patient had duodenal ulcers as well as
edema and dilatation of the duodenum and proximal

jejunum as shown in the barium x-ray clue. Steatorrhea may also occur since the low pH in the duodenum inactivates lipase.

5. Ultrasound, angiography (looking for tumor "blush") and CT scan each have about a 20% positive rate for pancreatic Z-E tumors. Their accuracy is approximately the same for liver metastases. If no obvious pancreatic mass is seen, transhepatic catheterization of the splenic vein, sampling areas in the pancreatic head, body and tail for serum gastrin, may provide a degree of tumor localization. Imaging studies were negative in this patient and transhepatic catheterization of the splenic vein was not performed.

6. The upper gastrointestinal inflammatory reaction should be treated with an H2-receptor antagonist. After healing has occurred and if no metastatic disease is apparent, the question of resectability should be considered. Although no tumor was identified by imaging studies, this patient underwent exploration after 8 weeks of medical therapy. Approximately 15% of such patients are found to have resectable pancreatic or extrapancreatic lesions, although no tumor was identified in this patient. A parietal cell vagotomy has been advised by some surgeons since it may decrease the required dose of H2-receptor antagonist. If metastatic disease is discovered before or during surgery, appropriate biopsies are obtained and chemotherapy (often including streptozocin) is begun. Long-term medical management with H2-receptor antagonists has been successful, provided that adequate acid suppression is achieved. Omeprazole, an experimental inhibitor of hydrogen-potassium-ATPase on the luminal surface of the parietal cell, has been extremely effective in inhibiting acid production in Z-E patients. A basal acid output less than 10 mEq/liter 1 hour before the next dose should be achieved. Total gastrectomy is reserved for those patients who find it difficult to take medication on a rigid schedule or who fail to respond to medical therapy.

PEARLS

1. In the previously unoperated patient, a serum gastrin of 1,000 pg/ml or higher, in the presence of gastric hypersecretion, is likely to reflect a Z-E syndrome and does not require a secretin provocative test.

2. The presence or absence of symptoms cannot be used to
    determine whether medical therapy is adequately
    suppressing gastric acid production, thus the need to
    check basal acid output prior to the next dose of a
    histamine-2 receptor antagonist.

3. If the gastric acid fails to respond to standard doses
    of a histamine-2 receptor antagonist, a trial of an
    anticholinergic should be considered before the
    H2-receptor antagonist dose is increased.

4. Although gastroduodenal ulcer disease is most commonly
    associated with the Z-E syndrome, patients may present
    with extremely severe gastroesophageal reflux disease.

5. Diarrhea may be severe in some patients with the Z-E
    syndrome. The symptom can be initially managed with
    nasogastric suction until pharmacologic control is
    achieved.

PITFALLS

1. Isolated tumors in the pancreatic head of a patient
    with Z-E syndrome should be enucleated, but
    pancreaticoduodenectomy should be avoided since
    extrapancreatic or multiple primaries may exist.

2. Sucralfate has no effect on gastric acid secretion and
    therefore has little value in the therapy of Z-E
    syndrome.

3. Do not proceed with abdominal surgery until
    parathyroidectomy has been performed in hypercalcemic
    patients with the Z-E syndrome.

4. A surgical approach to the Z-E syndrome in patients
    with MEA-1 syndrome has not proven helpful since cure
    of the extensive pancreatic islet cell disease is
    uncommon. Drug therapy has been advocated as the
    preferred approach by several groups.

SUGGESTED READINGS

Cherner JA, Doppman JL, Norton JA: Selective venous
    sampling for gastrin to localize gastrinomas. Ann Int
    Med 105:841,1986.

Maton PN, Miller DL, Doppman JL: Role of selective
    angiography in the management of patients with
    Zollinger-Ellison syndrome.   Gastroenterology
    92:913, 1987.
Vinik AI, Thompson N: Controversies in the management of
    Zollinger-Ellison syndrome.   Ann Int Med 105:956, 1986.
Wank SA, Doppman JL, Miller DL: Prospective study of the
    ability of computed axial tomography to localize
    gastrinomas in patients with Zollinger-Ellison
    syndrome.   Gastroenterology 92:905, 1987.
Wolfe MM, Jensen RT: Zollinger-Ellison syndrome: Current
    concepts in diagnosis and management.   N Engl J Med
    317:1200, 1987

CASE 7:   OBSTRUCTIVE JAUNDICE IN AN ALCOHOLIC

A 59-year-old man complains of diminished appetite and
nausea for 1 month. There has been no abdominal pain or
fever, but he has lost approximately 10 pounds. He has
taken no medications, other than occasional acetominophen
for arthritic symptoms. He describes a daily alcohol
intake of approximately 1 pint of whiskey with a 6-pack of
beer, but he has been drinking less in the past few weeks.
He reports an episode of hepatitis while serving in the
Army during the Korean war. He underwent an antrectomy and
Billroth's II anastomosis 10 years ago for peptic ulcer
disease. Physical examination shows no scleral icterus.
The liver measures 10 cm from the superior to the inferior
margin and the spleen is not enlarged. There are no
abdominal masses or tenderness and the rectal examination
is unremarkable.

BILIARY ULTRASOUND CLUE

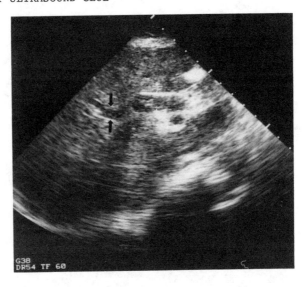

QUESTIONS (Please read the corresponding answer before proceeding to the next question.)

1. The presenting complaint of anorexia and nausea should orient you to which organ symptom?

2. What diagnostic possibilities should you consider?

3. The initial biochemical studies are as follows: bilirubin = 1.6 mg%; alkaline phosphatase = 190 units (normal to 85 units); AST (SGOT) = 93 units (normal to 40 units); ALT (SGPT) = 74 units (normal to 40 units); albumin = 4.3 g %; amylase = 115 units (normal to 100 units); lipase = 0.8 units (normal to 1.0 units), HBsAg negative, HBSAb negative. What information do you derive from this?

4. Does the negative HBsAg and HBsAb exclude hepatitis B disease?

5. What additional study would be most helpful?

6. Would you proceed with an endoscopic retrograde cholangiography (ERCP) or transhepatic cholangiogram?

7. How can a more specific diagnosis be established.

8. What approach would you now recommend?

ANSWERS

1. Anorexia and nausea are often considered
    "gastrointestinal symptoms," but these complaints can
    stem from disorders in any organ system as well as from
    drugs and emotional causes. Additional history,
    physical findings or laboratory studies usually will
    establish the specificity of these symptoms.

2. As indicated above, anorexia, nausea and weight loss
    could be due to a variety of disorders but his history
    suggests consideration of alcoholic liver disease,
    although one would expect hepatomegaly in the early
    phase. Alcoholic pancreatitis is more likely to
    produce pain before these more subtle symptoms are
    experienced. Alcoholic gastritis or peptic ulcer
    disease should be considered. The history of previous
    hepatitis raises the possibility of chronic hepatitis
    or cirrhosis, although there are no physical findings
    to support this. Finally, anorexia, nausea and weight
    loss in a 59-year-old man could be the result of an
    occult neoplasm.

3. Abnormal liver function tests rarely provide a specific
    diagnosis. The commonly ordered studies indicate
    whether there is an abnormality in bile secretion
    (cholestasis), bilirubin conjugation or uptake, or
    evidence of hepatocyte damage. This patient shows a
    high degree of cholestasis (alkaline phosphatase twice
    the top normal value) and moderate hepatocyte damage
    (acute viral hepatitis generally leads to transaminase
    levels 10 times the top normal value). The minimal
    elevation of amylase is not helpful at this point. The
    patient has an obstructive pattern of liver dysfunction
    and indicates the need to distinguish between hepatic
    and extrahepatic etiologies.

4. This patient could be in the serologic gap phase of
    hepatitis B disease, the period between return of the
    surface antigen to nonmeasurable levels and the
    appearance of the surface antibody, which takes several
    months. If this possibility is considered, the
    hepatitis B core antibody can be helpful. The IgM
    fraction indicates an acute process. The recent onset
    of symptoms in this patient suggests a beginning rather
    than resolving process.

5. An ultrasound study of the liver, biliary tract and
    pancreas would be the most direct approach. In this
    case it showed a common bile duct measuring 8 mm (see

arrow) with evidence of enlargement of the pancreatic head. The normal common bile duct is usually 5 mm or less, ducts between 5 and 7 mm are probably dilated, and over 7 mm is definitely enlarged. Patients with acute biliary obstruction may present with a normal common bile duct by ultrasound since there may not have been sufficient time for dilation. Cholescintography may show failure of the technetium 99-labeled iminodiacetic acid to enter the duodenum.

6. The approach to the biliary tract can be accomplished via the liver or by endoscopic retrograde cholangiography (ERCP), often depending upon the interests and experience of the hospital radiologists and gastroenterologists. This patient has had a Billroth's II anastomosis which increases the difficulty of ampullary cannulation. A transhepatic cholangiogram was performed which showed a narrowing of the distal common duct. A decompressing catheter was left in place. Although a smooth tapering of the distal duct suggests a benign etiology, such as pancreatitis, carcinoma may be difficult to exclude. We have also had experience in our institution with percutaneous injection of the gallbladder for the purpose of visualizing the biliary tract.

7. Percutaneous fine-needle aspiration of the pancreatic mass was performed during the cholangiogram, using the dye-filled bile duct as a guide. The cytologic biopsies showed evidence of adenocarcinoma.

8. A surgical approach should be considered for patients with pancreatic carcinoma if there is no evidence of metastasis. A CT scan showed the presence of peripancreatic node enlargement. The tumor also seemed a bit larger than was appreciated on the ultrasound study. A biliary stent was transhepatically inserted through the stenotic segment into the duodenum. No chemotherapy or radiation was offered.

PEARLS

1. Although obstruction of the common bile duct may result from acute pancreatitis, complete obstruction (clay-colored stools) is uncommon.

2. Alcoholic hepatitis may result in a classic picture of cholestatic liver disease, thus raising the possibility of extrahepatic obstruction.

3. Intermittent episodes of ascending cholangitis are more common with common bile duct stones than with malignant obstruction. This probably stems from the proliferation of bacteria trapped in the surface of the stone.

4. When considering malignant obstruction of the biliary tree, search carefully for a cholangiocarcinoma at the bifurcation of the common duct. Ultrasound or CT scan will show dilated intrahepatic bile ducts with a normal diameter common bile duct.

5. The presence of upper abdominal pain, epigastric bruit and splenomegaly should suggest the presence of segmental hypertension, pressure on the splenic vein and artery by pancreatic malignancy or pseudocyst.

6. Patients with pancreatic carcinoma presenting with painless jaundice have the best chance for surgical resectability and cure, although it was not possible in this patient.

PITFALLS

1. Determination of the direct and indirect bilirubin fractions is not useful in distinguishing between hepatic and extrahepatic jaundice. Bilirubin fractionation is best used for distinguishing between prehepatic (hemolysis, Gilbert's disease) and hepatic jaundice.

2. Patients operated on for biliary diversion secondary to common bile duct obstruction by a pancreatic mass must have operative cytologic biopsies of the pancreas as well as excision of surrounding nodes. It may be difficult for the surgeon to distinguish between pancreatitis and carcinoma since they may coexist.

3. If there is evidence of partial obstruction of the common bile duct during an acute episode of pancreatitis, it is safer to defer an ERCP until the acute process has subsided.

4. Fever in a patient with an internal biliary stent should always be considered cholangitis unless some other cause is readily apparent. Delay in obtaining blood cultures and starting broad spectrum antibiotic therapy could result in liver abscesses. The most common cause for infection is obstruction (66%) and the

organisms most often recovered from the blood are Escherichia coli and Pseudomonas aeruginosa, while the most common organisms recovered from the bile are Pseudomonas aeruginosa, Klebsiella pneumoniae and Streptococcus faecalis.

SUGGESTED READINGS

Bornman PC, Tobias R, Harries-Jones EP, et al: Prospective controlled trial of transhepatic biliary endoprosthesis versus bypass surgery for incurable carcinoma of head of pancreas. Lancet 1:69, 1986.

Dooley JS, Dick R, George P: Percutaneous transhepatic endoprosthesis for bile duct obstruction. Gastroenterology 86:905, 1984.

Malt RA: Treatment of pancreatic cancer. JAMA 250:1433, 1983.

Patwardhan RV, Smith OJ, Farmelant MH: Serum transaminase levels and cholescintigraphic abnormalities in acute biliary tract obstruction. Arch Intern Med 147:1249, 1987.

Speer AG, Russell RCG, Hatfield AR: Randomized trial of endoscopic versus percutaneous stent insertion in malignant obstructive jaundice. Lancet 2:57, 1987.

Szabo S, Mendelson MH, Mitty HA: Infections associated with transhepatic biliary drainage devices. Am J Med 82:921, 1987.

CASE 8:   LEFT LOWER QUADRANT PAIN AND BOWEL IRREGULARITY

A 49-year-old businesswoman has experienced occasional
bowel irregularity and abdominal discomfort but she now
presents with the complaint of increasing left lower
abdominal pain and constipation alternating with bouts of
diarrhea.   The pain varies from mild to very severe and may
last for hours.   Mucus has been seen covering the stool.
Belching and flatulence have been more prominent.   There
has been no rectal bleeding, fever or weight loss.   The
patient had travelled to Leningrad 1 month before symptoms
began.   She has been using a variety of analgesics and
laxatives.   Physical examination shows tenderness in the
left lower quadrant with no muscle guarding.   There is no
organ enlargement or abdominal bruit and the rectal
examination is unremarkable.   An office CBC is normal.

BARIUM ENEMA CLUE

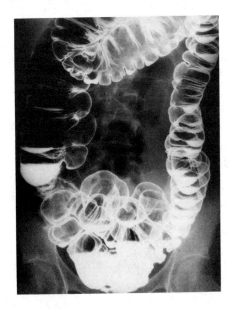

QUESTIONS (Please read the corresponding answer before proceeding to the next question.)

1. What is your differential diagnosis of left lower quadrant abdominal pain and tenderness?

2. What is the significance of the patient's travel history?

3. How important is the description of mucus with the stools?

4. What studies would your order?

5. Does intestinal gas play a role in the abdominal pain of patients with the irritable bowel syndrome?

6. Could lactase deficiency produce these symptoms?

7. What therapeutic program would you outline for this patient?

ANSWERS

1. Diverticulitis can cause left lower quadrant pain and
    tenderness. This patient has no fever or leukocytosis,
    thus making the diagnosis less likely. The possibility
    of an ovarian disorder prompted a gynecologic
    examination, which was unremarkable. Inflammatory
    bowel disease can cause lower abdominal pain,
    tenderness and diarrhea, but a normal flexible
    sigmoidoscopy to 55 cm reasonably excluded ulcerative
    and Crohn's colitis. A barium enema was obtained for
    better evaluation of the remaining colon and this was
    also normal (see Clue). The irritable bowel syndrome
    becomes increasingly likely in view of these normal
    findings. Left lower quadrant tenderness without
    muscle guarding or rebound tenderness (without fever or
    leukocytosis) supports this consideration.

2. Giardiasis is endemic in Leningrad. The symptoms
    include crampy abdominal pain, gaseousness and
    variable degrees of bowel irregularity. The stool
    examination for ova and parasites was negative, but a
    higher degree of concern would have prompted
    microscopic evaluation of duodenal juice for the
    parasites.

3. Increased colonic mucus production is found in some
    patients with the spastic colon form of the irritable
    bowel syndrome, thus the old terminology, "mucus
    colitis." Patients with colitis of any cause
    (ulcerative, Crohn's, parasitic, radiation) also pass
    secretions with the stool which resemble mucus, but
    microscopy often shows considerable quantities of white
    blood cells, indicating the presence of pus rather than
    pure mucus.

4. As indicated above, stool examinations for ova and
    parasites, sigmoidoscopy, barium enema, and upper GI
    barium study with small bowel examination would
    reasonably exclude an inflammatory disorder in the mid
    and lower intestinal tract.

5. Intestinal wash-out techniques show that patients
    usually have less than 200 cc of gas in the small and
    large bowel at any time, with no clear-cut difference
    between normals and those with the irritable bowel
    syndrome. Nevertheless, the infusion of gas into the
    proximal duodenum elicits considerably more discomfort
    in those with an irritable bowel than in normals,
    suggesting a greater degree of sensitivity to

distension in the functional group. This same effect can be shown by inflating balloons in the colon of normal and irritable bowel patients.

6. Although lactase deficiency is often considered to produce diarrhea in milk-drinking patients, some individuals present with crampy pain and flatulence.

7. a. The thorough evaluation, reviewing the negative findings with the patient, can serve to allay the anxiety that some patients have about persisting abdominal complaints.
b. Dietary instructions need not be rigorous, but efforts to reduce swallowed air can be helpful, such as eliminating carbonated beverages and sucking on hard candies. Roughage, such as fruit, salad, and bran, should be avoided if diarrhea is prominent, but can be added when constipation is a problem.
c. Anticholinergic medications can be used if pain is a predominant feature, providing that there are no contraindications, such as glaucoma, prostate disease or cardiac disorders. This approach can lead to increased constipation, thus the need to add roughage, perhaps with the use of a psyllium product and stool softeners. Occasional loperamide or Lomotil (generic) can be used to control episodes of diarrhea, but should not be given chronically.

PEARLS

1. The location of abdominal pain in irritable bowel patients need not indicate the segment of bowel responsible for the discomfort, since inflation of a balloon in the hepatic or splenic flexure of the colon could induce pain in the lower quadrants.

2. Insufflation of air into the colon during sigmoidoscopy or barium enema may reproduce the pain experienced by an irritable bowel patient.

3. The complaint of flatulence may reflect the patient's fastidiousness and current interest. It may be helpful to ask the patient to keep a diary of the number of gas passages per day. Since normal young adults have approximately 14 plus or minus 4 passages per day, the record keeping may serve to reassure some patients that their "excessive" flatulence is a normal phenomenon.

4. The diarrheal phase of the irritable colon is usually
    not associated with significant pain, does not awaken
    the patient from sleep and is most troublesome in the
    morning.

5. Although diabetic patients may also experience
    recurrent constipation or diarrhea, the associated
    sphincter disturbances (bowel and/or bladder),
    peripheral neuropathy or retinal findings should
    establish the diagnosis of autonomic neuropathy.

PITFALLS

1. Patients with functional gastrointestinal symptoms
    should not be referred for psychiatric help unless a
    clear-cut emotional disorder is present. Many patients
    perceive this as a message from their physician that
    the symptoms are purely from "nerves" or that the pain
    is "imaginary." Although tensional factors may
    influence these symptoms, malfunction of the intestinal
    tract often plays an important role.

2. Rectal gas should not be solely ascribed to swallowed
    air since colonic production of hydrogen and carbon
    dioxide from unabsorbed dietary carbohydrate may
    contribute, in varying degrees, to total gas output.

3. Do not use oral narcotics for the treatment of patients
    with chronic functional abdominal pain. Addiction is
    likely and the constipation becomes more severe.

4. Avoid providing detailed, rigorous diet sheets to
    patients with the irritable bowel syndrome. These
    bland (tasteless) or low roughage instructions are
    difficult to follow and give the patient another layer
    of concern and, eventually, frustration.

5. Do not suggest to a patient with chronic functional
    symptoms that any therapeutic regimen is "curative,"
    since these disorders tend to be recurrent. The
    patient might be instructed to follow the medications
    and dietary suggestions while symptomatic and then stop
    therapy when comfortable, with the understanding that
    treatment will be resumed when symptoms return.

SUGGESTED READINGS

Creed R, Guthrie E: Psychological factors in the irritable
    bowel syndrome. Gut 28:1307, 1987.
Meunier P: Physiologic study of the terminal digestive
    tract in chronic painful constipation. Gut 27:1018,
    1986.
Rose JDR, Troughton AH, Harvey JS, et al: Depression and
    functional bowel disorders in gastrointestinal
    outpatients. Gut 27:1025, 1986.
Stokes MA, Moriarty KJ, Catchpole BN: A study of the
    genesis of colic. Lancet 1:211, 1988.
Swarbrick ET, Bat L, Hegarty JE, et al: Site of pain from
    the irritable bowel. Lancet 2:443, 1980.
Thompson WG: A strategy for management of the irritable
    bowel. Am J Gastroenterol 81:95, 1986.

CASE 9: LEFT LOWER QUADRANT PAIN AND FEVER

A 71-year-old woman had been in reasonably good health
until she began to experience intermittent fevers to 101 F
associated with lower abdominal discomfort. Occasional
loose stools were reported without evidence of gross
bleeding. She became anorexic but did not vomit. Symptoms
persisted for 1 week and eventuated in admission to
hospital. Her chest and heart were normal. The abdomen
showed mild lower abdominal tenderness, somewhat more
marked in the left lower quadrant, without muscle guarding.
Bowel sounds were normal. A rectal examination showed soft
brown stool which was negative for occult blood. The
hemoglobin was 12.5 g%, white blood count 12,400 with 83
segs, 14 lymphs and 3 monos. The urinalysis showed 8-10
red blood cells per high-power field.

BARIUM ENEMA CLUE

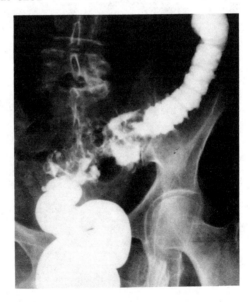

QUESTIONS (Please read the corresponding answer before proceeding to the next question.)

1. What diagnoses would you consider?

2. What studies would you initially order?

3. Would colonoscopy be of value at this point?

4. Would you start antibiotics at this point?

5. What is the risk of deferring antibiotic therapy?

6. When would you order a barium enema?

7. Should you operate on this patient?

ANSWERS

1. Although the irritable bowel syndrome can produce
    crampy abdominal pain, the presence of fever and
    leukocytosis in an elderly patient with no previous
    history of bowel disease reasonably excludes this
    consideration.

    Fever, abdominal pain and left lower quadrant
    tenderness should suggest diverticulitis, particularly
    if the patient is over 50 years of age. Crohn's
    disease, however, has been known to occur in the older
    age group (so-called "second-peak") and ischemic
    colitis should be considered in the older patient. A
    confined perforation of a sigmoid colon carcinoma could
    produce an identical clinical picture. Infectious
    colitis, such as Campylobacter, might be considered,
    but this patient had no diarrhea and the stool was
    negative for occult blood.

2. a. An obstruction series would be useful in order to
    determine if there was evidence of partial or complete
    bowel obstruction or air within an abscess cavity. The
    x-ray was negative in this patient. Some patients
    present with small bowel obstructive signs and symptoms
    since the mid-ileum may be in close proximity to a
    sigmoid inflammatory reaction.
    b. Since diverticulitis is one of the considerations,
    an ultrasound of the left lower quadrant should be
    considered. It was also negative in this patient (as
    was a CT of the abdomen obtained several days later).
    c. Blood cultures should be obtained. (In this case
    they showed no growth.)
    d. If the patient was in a younger age group, a
    gynecologic examination would be indicated to rule out
    a ruptured ovarian cyst or pelvic inflammatory disease
    (PID).
    e. You might consider stool examinations for culture,
    sensitivity, ova and parasites.

3. Colonoscopy or flexible sigmoidoscopy should not be
    performed until the acute inflammatory reaction has
    subsided.

4. The presumptive diagnosis of diverticulitis is
    sufficient to begin broad spectrum antibiotic therapy
    designed for aerobic and anaerobic organisms, after
    blood cultures are obtained. A combination of
    gentamycin and clindamycin was begun.

5. Untreated diverticulitis may lead to the spread of organisms to the portal system, causing pylephlebitis and/or hepatic abscesses, potentially lethal complications.

6. The barium enema should be deferred until there is evidence of improvement in the inflammatory reaction. The study was obtained in this patient after 7 days of clear liquids and antibiotics. It was performed without air insufflation and showed evidence of sigmoid diverticula, narrowing in the sigmoid colon, and extrinsic pressure on the sigmoid suggesting the presence of a pericolonic mass (see Clue).

7. The patient clinically responded to antibiotic therapy, the fever and leukocytosis normalized, and she subsequently tolerated a full diet without difficulty. She has a 50% chance of not experiencing a recurrent episode of diverticulitis, so that elective surgery should not be performed. However, failure to respond to the therapy, unremitting bowel obstruction or other complications might have prompted a diverting colosotomy with resection of the involved sigmoid, or one-stage resection and anastomosis, depending on the surgical findings.

PEARLS

1. Acute diverticulitis is not generally associated with gross rectal bleeding. Conversely, brisk bleeding from a colonic diverticulum is not usually accompanied by signs of diverticulitis (fever, localized tenderness and leukocytosis).

2. There are many similarities between appendicitis and diverticulitis, including early visceral pain, nausea and vomiting, and shifting pain and tenderness. If the sigmoid colon is redundant and lies in the right lower quadrant, the distinction between the 2 disorders may be extremely difficult.

3. The radiographic diagnosis of diverticulitis requires the presence of an extrinsic mass, fistula or obstruction associated with diverticula. Milder forms of diverticulitis may not be detected.

4. Acute diverticulitis usually extends beyond the confines of the colon (as do the diverticula), but some

cases have an inflammatory reaction localized to the wall of the colon (intramural diverticulitis).

5. The passage of gas with urination (pneumaturia) usually indicates the presence of a colovesicle fistula. The symptom should be specifically sought since patients may not volunteer the information. Colovesical fistulas are less common in women because of the interposed uterus.

PITFALLS

1. Although pneumaturia may be absent, the presence of diverticulitis adjacent to the bladder may produce urinary findings consistent with cystitis.

2. Colonoscopy performed during the active phase of diverticulitis is hazardous since distension of the colon may cause perforation of the inflammatory reaction.

3. Although it is preferable to defer a contrast study of the colon during acute diverticulitis, if circumstances require an imaging examination, such as the need to distinguish between appendicitis and diverticulitis, it would be well to avoid barium. If extravasated, barium causes considerably more problems in the peritoneal cavity than gastrografin. The contrast enema is superior to CT for the diagnosis of diverticulitis, although the latter may be considered if an abscess is suspected and not conclusively shown by the contrast study. An ultrasound could also be used for the same purpose.

4. One-stage resection and reanastomosis of the left colon for diverticulitis should only be attempted if the entire inflammatory reaction can be removed without any residual bacterial contamination or significant inflammatory reaction. It is always safer, if any question of the status of the operative field exists, to remove the inflamed sigmoid and perform a diverting colostomy, with reanastomosis at a later date.

5. Although the x-rays and clinical picture, in some cases, may indicate diverticulitis, a perforated or obstructing carcinoma may mimic diverticulitis so closely that the surgeon may have difficulty in distinguishing between the two diseases.

SUGGESTED READINGS

Frager D, Wolf EL, Beneventano TC: Small intestinal
    complications of diverticulitis of the sigmoid colon.
    JAMA 256:3258, 1986.
Johnson CD, Baker ME, Rice RP, et al: Diagnosis of acute
    colonic diverticulitis: Comparison of barium enema and
    CT.   Am J Radiol 148:541, 1987.
Krukowski ZH, Koruth NM, Matheson NA: Evolving practice in
    acute diverticulitis.   Br J Surg 72:684, 1985.
Silen, W: Cope's Early Diagnosis of the Acute Abdomen, ed.
    17.   New York, Oxford University Press, 1987, pp
    100-101.

CASE 10:   ASCITES AND LIVER DYSFUNCTION

A 34-year-old woman with a 10-year history of heavy alcohol
intake is admitted with the complaint of increasing
abdominal girth of 2 weeks duration. She had been
diagnosed by liver biopsy as having cirrhosis 18 months
ago. She has mild abdominal discomfort. Her vital signs
are normal. There has been no obvious gastrointestinal
bleeding. Physical examination shows muscle wasting and
tense abdominal distension with shifting dullness. She has
spider nevi on the upper chest. Liver and spleen size are
difficult to determine with confidence, due to the ascites.
Mild tenderness is present. There is no peripheral edema.
A digital rectal examination is negative. The hemoglobin
is 10.2 g%, white blood count is 4,900 and the platelet
count is 89,000.

CLUE

The ascitic fluid albumin is 1.9 g%, the serum albumin is
3.3 g% and the ascites white blood count is 178.

QUESTIONS (Please read the corresponding answer before proceeding to the next question.)

1. How can you best determine if this patient has spontaneous bacterial peritonitis?

2. How can you determine whether the ascitic fluid is a "transudate" or "exudate"?

3. What dietary and pharmacologic approach would you begin with?

4. Does the presence of peripheral edema influence your therapy?

5. Although this patient began to respond to medical therapy, what strategies would you consider if no diuresis was achievable?

ANSWERS

1. A needle paracentesis is essential to evaluate the
    possibility of spontaneous bacterial peritonitis
    because of her abdominal tenderness. The absence of
    fever and leukocytosis does not rule out the
    possibility. An ascites white blood count count less
    than 300 cells/cc reasonably excludes spontaneous
    bacterial peritonitis. The ascites pH and lactate have
    also been used for this purpose but are less sensitive.
    If the white blood count count is over 1,000, broad
    spectrum antibiotics should be started until the
    culture results are available.

2. The specific gravity and protein content have generally
    been used to distinguish between the ascites derived
    from portal hypertension ("transudate") and fluid from
    inflammatory or neoplastic causes ("exudate"). This is
    not a reliable approach since 19% of patients with
    cirrhotic ascites have been reported to have a high
    ascitic protein content. A more helpful strategy is to
    subtract the ascites albumin from the serum albumin.
    If the difference is less than 1.1 g%, it is likely to
    be inflammatory or exudative, while values greater than
    1.1 g% are consistent with ascites secondary to portal
    hypertension.

3. Diet: Sodium, 250-500 mg/day. Fluid need not be
    stringently restricted unless the serum sodium is below
    130 mEq/liter. If this occurs, fluid should be
    restricted to approximately 1,000 cc/day.

    Drugs: A potassium-sparing diuretic, such as
    spironolactone (100-600 mg/day) or Dyrenium, should be
    given. The dose should be increased until diuresis
    occurs. If there if no response, a loop diuretic such
    as furosemide should be added in increasing doses.

4. Studies have suggested that approximately 300 cc can
    be absorbed from the peritoneal cavity in 24 hours
    during diuretic therapy in the absence of peripheral
    edema and approximately 900 cc in the presence of
    peripheral edema. More recent work suggests that
    somewhat larger volumes can be mobilized, so that a
    diuresis of 0.75 kg/day in the absence of peripheral
    edema and greater than 2 kg/day can be accomplished if
    peripheral edema is present.

5. Some patients with tense ascites do not respond to
    large doses of spironolactone (400-800 mg/day) and

furosemide (120 mg/day or greater). It is important to ascertain whether the patient is surreptitiously taking salt or excess fluids. The intravenous infusion of salt-poor albumin has been advocated but the response to this approach is not generally satisfactory. Large volume paracentesis (3-6 liters over 4-6 hours) in addition to intravenous salt-poor albumin (approximately 10 g for every liter of ascites removed) can provide a measure of comfort and perhaps prevent reaccumulation of the ascites in conjunction with the diuretic program outlined in answer 4. Large-volume paracentesis may be required if tense ascites causes respiratory difficulty. If, however, fluid does recur, consideration should be given to a peritoneal-jugular shunt.

PEARLS

1. Physical examination techniques can demonstrate the presence of approximately 500-1000 ml of free intra-abdominal fluid. Ultrasound is capable of detecting as little as 100 cc of free fluid.

2. The presence of an ascitic fluid lactic dehydrogenase (LDH) significantly higher than the serum LDH should suggest malignant ascites. The fluid should also be sent for cytologic examination.

3. Malignant ascites generally does not respond as well as cirrhotic ascites to diuretic therapy. Such patients may be candidates for a peritoneal-jugular shunt. The procedure should not be performed if the protein content exceeds 3 g%, since viscid fluid may "clog" the shunt tubing.

4. It is difficult to restrict oral fluids for many hospitalized patients. One strategy is to instruct the patient that every container of fluid is counted as "1" and that the patient is entitled to 6 (or more) containers per day (juice, coffee, water, etc.), assuming approximately 200 cc per container.

PITFALLS

1. Needle paracentesis should not be performed through or near an abdominal incisional scar since bowel loops may be adhesed to the anterior abdominal wall. Be certain that the patient voids prior to paracentesis. (You do

not wish to find a report of "casts" in your specimen.)
Coagulation studies should be checked prior to the
procedure since serious complications can occur.

2. Do not prescribe routine potassium supplements to
    patients receiving potassium-sparing drugs.
    Hyperkalemia may well result.

3. It is unnecessary to prompt diuresis in an ascitic
    patient to the point of dryness. The risk of
    dehydration and electrolyte imbalance clearly rise in
    the presence of overly aggressive therapy. A modest
    amount of ascites is not a medical threat.

4. Nonsteroidal anti-inflammatory drugs should not be used
    in patients with cirrhotic ascites since prostaglandin
    inhibition reduces renal function in such patients.

5. Only 5% of patients with cirrhotic ascites fail to
    respond to appropriate medical therapy. The
    peritoneal-jugular shunt should be reserved for this
    group. The procedure has a significant complication
    rate with an operative mortality as high as 3%, and the
    mortality in the 1st month may approach 25%. Shunt
    failure occurs in approximately 10% of cases.

SUGGESTED READINGS

Attali P, Turner K, Pelletier G, et al: pH of ascitic
    fluid: Diagnostic and prognostic value in cirrhotic
    and noncirrhotic patients. Gastroenterology
    90:1255, 1986.
Gines P, Arroyo V, Quintero E, et al: Comparison of
    paracentesis and diuretics in the treatment of
    cirrhotics with tense ascites. Gastroenterology
    93:234, 1987.
Pockros PJ, Reynolds TB: Rapid diuresis in patients with
    ascites from chronic liver disease: The importance of
    peripheral edema. Gastroenterology 90:1827, 1986.
Rector WG: An improved diagnostic approach to ascites.
    Arch Intern Med 147:215, 1987.
Rocco VK, Ware AJ: Cirrhotic ascites: Pathophysiology,
    diagnosis, and management. Ann Int Med 105:573, 1986.
Rubinstein D, Mcinnes I, Dudley F: Morbidity and mortality
    after peritoneovenous shunt surgery for refractory
    ascites. Gut 26:1070, 1985.

CASE 11:   CHRONIC ULCERATIVE COLITIS AND ANEMIA

A 32-year-old woman developed the onset of severe ulcerative colitis at age 14, requiring several hospital admissions over a 3-year period. Her disease at that time involved the entire colon. She eventually responded to medical therapy and was maintained on low-dose prednisone and sulfasalazine for several years, with adjustment of dosage depending on disease activity. Her symptoms became progressively less severe over the years until 6 weeks prior to admission, when rectal bleeding became more prominent and she became somewhat fatigued. Physical examination showed no abdominal tenderness or organ enlargement. The hemoglobin was 9.2 g%, white blood count 7,900 with a normal differential count.

BARIUM ENEMA CLUE

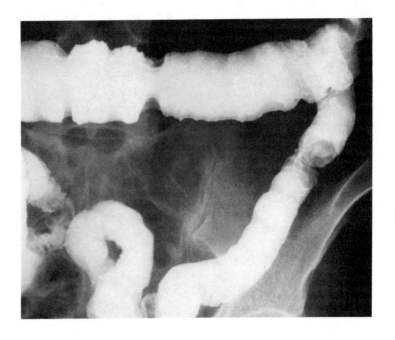

QUESTIONS (Please read the corresponding answer before proceeding to the next question.)

1. What is your differential diagnosis?

2. What studies will be most helpful in establishing the diagnosis?

3. How could this complication have been prevented?

ANSWERS

1. a. This could be an exacerbation of her ulcerative
    colitis.
    b. She may have a superimposed bacterial colitis, such
    as Campylobacter.
    c. The rectal bleeding and anemia could be the result
    of adenocarcinoma.

2. a. Stool cultures and examinations for ova and
    parasites. (These were negative.)
    b. Flexible sigmoidoscopy. In this case the
    examination was performed to 30 cm and showed very mild
    granularity without mucosal bleeding, although some
    blood was seen coming from "above." Active ulcerative
    colitis almost always involves the rectum, so that the
    mild changes seen in this case suggest pathology higher
    in the sigmoid or left colon. A colonoscopic
    examination showed a polypoid mass in the descending
    colon which proved to be adenocarcinoma; the mass was
    also shown by barium enema (see Clue).

3. Patients with a history of severe ulcerative colitis of
    8-10 years duration should have yearly colonoscopic
    examinations to determine if early cancer can be
    identified, and colon biopsies to search for evidence
    of epithelial dysplasia. Severe dysplasia, marked
    branching or budding of the tubules with evidence of
    villous proliferation, indicates the need to repeat the
    examination in several months. If positive, the
    patient has an increased risk of having colon cancer
    (not identified by colonoscopy), or developing a
    malignancy. Prophylactic colectomy should be
    considered, with end ileostomy, continent ileostomy or
    a sphincter-preserving procedure and construction of a
    "J-pouch."

PEARLS

1. Carcinoma is more likely to develop if the entire colon
    (or at least 1/2 the colon) has been involved at some
    time. Patients with long-standing proctosigmoiditis
    are at considerably less risk. Unfortunately, the
    precise risk of carcinoma developing in patients with
    extensive ulcerative colitis has not been determined
    with confidence, but clearly exceeds that found in the
    general population.

2. There is no correlation between the degree of colitis activity and the likelihood of dysplasia (or malignancy) at the time the biopsy is performed. The patient may be in complete remission and have biopsy evidence of advanced dysplasia.

3. Carcinomas in ulcerative colitis differ from those found in otherwise normal patients in the following manner:
    a. There is no predilection for the rectosigmoid area. The tumors can be found anywhere in the colon.
    b. Ulcerative colitis patients are usually a decade younger than other patients with carcinoma.
    c. There is a higher incidence of multiple primary carcinomas in colitis patients.
    d. There is a higher frequency of poorly differentiated adenocarcinomas.

4. Patients who undergo a colectomy for severe epithelial dysplasia may be found to have a carcinoma which was not detected by barium enema or colonoscopy.

PITFALLS

1. The pain and bleeding experienced by colitis patients lead to a longer delay in cancer diagnosis since both patient and physician may interpret the symptoms as reflecting colitis activity.

2. The barium enema is not as reliable as colonoscopy for the purpose of determining the extent of colitis activity. For instance, if the barium enema shows evidence of colitis extending to the distal transverse colon, colonoscopy often shows involvement of the entire colon.

3. The diagnosis of epithelial dysplasia is a difficult one. It is prudent to obtain a second opinion by an established authority in the field before subjecting a patient to prophylactic colectomy.

4. Although early reports suggested that rectal biopsies were sufficient for the diagnosis of dysplasia in chronic ulcerative colitis, it is apparent that dysplasia is often patchy and may spare the rectum. Biopsies, therefore, must be obtained from all portions of the colon and particularly from any sessile lesions, since dysplasia from the surface of a small mass or nodule is often found to be associated with carcinoma.

SUGGESTED READINGS

Brostrom O, Lofberg R, Ost A, et al: Cancer surveillance
    of patients with longstanding ulcerative colitis: A
    clinical, endoscopical, and histological study. Gut
    27:1408, 1986.
Collins RH, Feldman M, Fordtran JS: Colon cancer,
    dysplasia, and surveillance in patients with ulcerative
    colitis: A critical review. N Engl J Med 316:1654,
    1987.
Katzka I, Brody RS, Morris E, et al: Assessment of
    colorectal cancer risk in patients with ulcerative
    colitis: Experience from a private practice.
    Gastroenterology 85:22, 1987.
Lashner BA, Hanauer SB, Silverstein MD: Optimal timing of
    colonoscopy to screen for cancer in ulcerative colitis.
    Ann Int Med 108:274, 1988.
Lennard-Jones JE: Compliance, cost, and common sense limit
    cancer control in colitis. Gut 27:1403, 1986.
Morson BC, Pang LSC: Rectal biopsy as an aid to cancer
    control in ulcerative colitis. Gut 8:423, 1967.

CASE 12: CHEST PAIN AND A NEGATIVE CARDIAC EVALUATION

A 53-year-old hospital administrator presented to his internist with the complaint of intermittent episodes of mid and low substernal chest discomfort over a 6-week period. The pain seemed unrelated to exertion, did not radiate to his back or shoulders and was described as a "pressure" sensation. Physical examination showed no abnormality of the chest or abdomen. The patient experienced occasional heartburn but denied dysphagia. A complete cardiac evaluation, including stress testing and thallium imaging was unremarkable.

ESOPHAGEAL MOTILITY CLUE

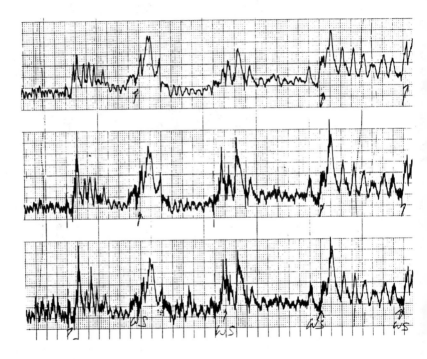

QUESTIONS (Please read the corresponding answer before proceeding to the next question.)

1. a. What percentage of patients with angina-like symptoms is found to have a normal cardiac evaluation?

    b. What percentage of patients with noncardiac angina is found to have an esophageal etiology?

2. What studies would you obtain at this point?

3. How would you distinguish diffuse esophageal spasm from the "nutcracker esophagus" by esophageal manometry? Which is the more common cause for noncardiac chest pain?

4. If the esophageal motility study is normal, is there a strategy for reproducing a motility disorder in patients with noncardiac chest pain?

5. What treatment can be offered for this patient?

ANSWERS

1. a. Ten to 30% of patients with angina-like chest pain
        fail to show evidence of cardiac disease.
    b. Approximately 50-75% of patients with noncardiac
        chest pain are found to have an esophageal etiology.
        Disorders such as diffuse esophageal spasm, "nutcracker
        esophagus," hypertensive lower esophageal sphincter,
        vigorous achalasia, reflux esophagitis and carcinoma
        should be considered.

2. Consider the following studies:
    a. Bernstein test to determine if the dilute acid
        (0.1 N HCl) reproduces the patient's pain. (It was
        negative in this patient.)
    b. An isotope transit time study of the esophagus.
        Although it was not performed in this patient, the
        transit time is usually delayed in the presence of most
        esophageal motility disorders.
    c. Esophageal motility study. The study showed
        simultaneous contractions consistent with diffuse
        esophageal spasm (see Clue).

3. The characteristic motility finding in diffuse
    esophageal spasm is simultaneous contractions.
    Ordinarily, peristalsis proceeds down the esophagus in
    an orderly and progressive fashion. The occurrence of
    simultaneous contractions indicates the presence of
    spasm. Peristalsis in the "nutcracker esophagus"
    proceeds sequentially and normally, but the amplitude
    of the contraction exceeds 180-200 mm Hg, thus
    presumably contributing to the chest pain. This
    patient had manometric evidence of "nutcracker
    esophagus". Diffuse esophageal spasm may also be
    demonstrated by barium upper GI x-ray (corkscrew
    esophagus), but this is an insensitive approach and
    many asymptomatic patients have radiographic evidence
    of esophageal spasm. The most convincing esophageal
    motility findings would be a motility disorder detected
    while the patient is having pain.

4. Motility abnormalities may be intermittent and should
    be associated with chest pain before a causal
    relationship is inferred. A search for a useful
    provocative test has led to the use of ergonovine, but
    the coronary risk of the procedure obviates its use.
    An edrophonium-provocative test is safer and has been
    used for the same purpose, but only approximately 30%
    of patients with esophageal spasm or "nutcracker
    esophagus" will have both chest pain and a motility

disorder demonstrated. The mechanism for its action in esophageal motility disorders is unknown.

5. The most important contribution of diagnostic studies for patients with noncardiac chest pain is the establishment of a diagnosis. Although esophageal motility disorders are not curable, the patient usually benefits from knowing what process is producing the symptoms. Calcium channel antagonists, such as nifedipine, decrease lower esophageal sphincter pressure and also reduce distal esophageal contraction pressures. Studies have shown that the high peristaltic pressures in the distal esophagus can be lowered by nifedipine, but this manometric improvement may not be accompanied by clinical improvement. Such therapy should be given a trial (it did not work for this patient) and sublingual nitrates may also be given (no improvement in this patient). The reassurance was probably the most important achievement of the investigation.

PEARLS

1. A "positive" Bernstein test (acid perfusion of the esophagus) usually reflects esophagitis secondary to gastroesophageal reflux, but the test could produce chest pain in patients with esophagitis resulting from other causes, such as monilia, viral infections (Herpes, cytomegalovirus (CMV)) or carcinoma.

2. Patients with substernal chest pain and dysphagia should have an upper GI barium x-ray or endoscopy to evaluate the possibility of luminal disease, such as carcinoma, stricture from reflux esophagitis or lower esophageal ring.

3. Patients with symptomatic diffuse esophageal spasm are more likely to experience dysphagia (sometimes in the absence of pain) than patients with the "nutcracker esophagus."

4. Occasional patients with diffuse esophageal spasm may experience some benefit from esophageal dilatation.

PITFALLS

1. Although a patient's chest discomfort may seem like esophageal spasm, begin the evaluation with a thorough

cardiac investigation. Patients are not likely to die suddenly from esophageal motility disorders.

2. The "nutcracker esophagus" is characterized by high-amplitude contractions and substernal chest discomfort. Some normal individuals, however, may have similar but asymptomatic motility findings.

3. Esophageal motility studies have not been a very useful diagnostic tool for noncardiac chest pain unless a provocative test is performed (see above).

SUGGESTED READINGS

Castell DO, Richter JE: Edrophonium testing for esophageal pain. Dig Dis Sci 32:897, 1987.
Chobanian SJ, Benjamin SB, Curtis DJ, et al: Systematic esophageal evaluation of patients with noncardiac chest pain. Arch Intern Med 146:1505, 1986.
Clouse RE, Eckert TC: Gastrointestinal symptoms of patients with esophageal contraction abnormalities. Dig Dis Sci 31:236, 1986.
DeCaestecker JS, Blackwell JN, Brown J, et al: The oesophagus as a cause of recurrent chest pain: Which patients should be investigated and which tests should be used? Lancet 2:1143, 1985.
Janssens J, Vantrappen G, Ghillebert G: 24-hour recording of esophageal pressure and pH in patients with noncardiac chest pain. Gastroenterology 90:1978, 1986.
Richter JE, Dalton CB, Bradley LA, et al: Oral nifedipine in the treatment of noncardiac chest pain in patients with the nutcracker esophagus. Gastroenterology 93:21, 1987.
Weinstock LB, Clouse RE: Esophageal physiology: Normal and abnormal motor function. Am J Gastroenterol 82:399, 1987.

CASE 13: DIARRHEA, CRAMPY PAIN AND WEIGHT LOSS

A 47-year-old woman presented with a 2-year history of diarrhea, crampy abdominal discomfort and fatigue. She had previously been in reasonably good health. She experienced 2 to 4 daily stools, varying from soft to liquid, associated with excessive flatulence. There had been a 12-pound weight loss since the onset of symptoms. The patient considered herself as "tense," owing to significant family problems. She had been treated with various antispasmodic and sedative medications without improvement. Upper and lower gastrointestinal barium x-rays were performed 18 months ago and were described as normal. She appeared somewhat malnourished, the abdominal examination was unremarkable, and the stool was negative for occult blood. The hemoglobin was 10.6 g%, mean corpuscular volume (MCV) 72, serum iron 45 ug/dL with a total iron binding capacity of 345 ug/dL, total protein of 6.5 g/dL and an albumin of 2.8 g/dL.

SMALL BOWEL BIOPSY CLUE

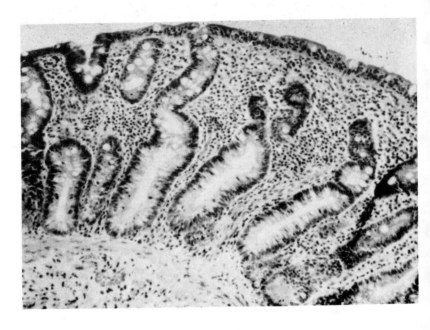

QUESTIONS (Please read the corresponding answer before proceeding to the next question.)

1. What diagnoses would you consider?

2. Should gastrointestinal x-rays be repeated?

3. What is the most sensitive study for the detection of steatorrhea?

4. How could you determine whether she has a problem with digestion or absorption?

5. What would be your next study to establish the diagnosis?

6. How can you be sure of your diagnosis?

ANSWERS

1. a. An irritable bowel syndrome could explain her
   symptoms, but weight loss, anemia and hypoalbuminemia
   would not be consistent with that diagnosis.
   b. Inflammatory bowel disease, particularly Crohn's
   disease, could account for her symptoms.
   c. Nontropical sprue. (Is she too old?)
   d. Tropical sprue. (She had no travel history to
   suggest this.)
   e. Lymphoma of the small bowel.
   f. Parasitic disorders (giardiasis, strongyloidiasis,
   hookworm).
   g. Chronic pancreatitis.

2. An upper gastrointestinal x-ray usually studies the
   esophagus, stomach and duodenum. The symptoms
   described in this case suggest the possibility of small
   bowel disease. An upper GI barium x-ray with small
   bowel follow-through (progress meal) was performed. It
   showed excess secretions and slight dilatation of the
   mucosal folds in the proximal small bowel. Stools for
   ova and parasites were obtained _prior_ to the x-ray
   study since barium interferes with the microscopic
   evaluation.

3. A stool microscopy with Sudan staining may demonstrate
   the presence of fat, but significant steatorrhea (over
   12-14 g/day) is usually required before the test is
   positive. A 3-day stool collection for the chemical
   determination of fat content remains the most sensitive
   available study for the determination of steatorrhea.
   If the patient is taking a diet of 100 g of fat daily
   during the collection period, excretion of over 7 g/day
   is considered abnormal (over 7% fecal excretion of
   the daily dietary fat intake). This patient's daily
   fat output was 13 g.

4. A D-xylose absorption test determines whether this
   pentose sugar is absorbed normally in the proximal
   small intestine. After a 25 g oral dose, this
   patient's urinary output was 2.3 g in 5 hours (normal
   over 5 g). Low excretion could also result from renal
   insufficiency, ascites, small bowel bacterial
   overgrowth, or delayed gastric emptying. Having
   determined that the proximal small bowel mucosal
   function was abnormal, a vitamin B-12 absorption test
   (Schilling test) was performed to evaluate the distal
   small bowel function (low excretion could result from
   pernicious anemia, small bowel bacterial overgrowth or

distal small bowel mucosal disease). The urinary
excretion of the isotope was normal. If the D-xylose
study had been normal, a secretin stimulation test of
pancreatic function would have been ordered to
determine if the steatorrhea resulted from a disorder
of digestion.

5. A small bowel biopsy was performed. This showed severe
mucosal atrophy, inflammatory changes and elongation of
the crypts of the distal duodenal mucosa consistent
with a diagnosis of sprue (or adult celiac disease).

6. The biopsy was consistent with sprue but a response to
a gluten-free diet is required to secure the diagnosis.
The patient's symptoms gradually subsided with close
adherence to the diet.

PEARLS

1. Dermatitis herpetiformis may occur in patients with
celiac disease, and a majority of such patients show
improvement or resolution of the skin disorder when
placed on a gluten-free diet.

2. The presence of an "oil slick" in the toilet bowel of
patients with steatorrhea is suggestive of the presence
of neutral fat, which should prompt consideration of
chronic pancreatitis (inability to split neutral fat
into fatty acids and monoglycerides). Steatorrhea may
be secondary to inadequate pancreatic enzyme secretion
in sprue patients as a result of inadequate
cholecystokinin release from the duodenum.

3. The anemia associated with sprue may be microcytic
secondary to the inability to absorb iron (as in this
patient), macroycytic secondary to folate deficiency or
"dimorphic" if both deficiencies are present.

4. Although the mucosa in celiac disease is often referred
to as "atrophic," the crypts are elongated and show
considerable mitotic activity. The flattened
epithelium represents a loss of surface epithelium in
excess of the ability of the crypts to synthesize new
cells. Celiac mucosa produces 6 times more cells per
hour than does normal mucosa.

5. Although the various small bowel suction biopsies
provide larger samples, multiple samples can also be

obtained via endoscopic examination of the distal 2nd portion of the duodenum.

PITFALLS

1. A response to a gluten-free diet is required to support the histologic and clinical impression of celiac disease, but failure to improve may represent poor compliance with the diet rather than an incorrect diagnosis. Improvement in symptoms may occur in 48 hours, but full remission may take weeks or months.

2. Both carcinoma (which may occur in the esophagus, pharynx, stomach and rectum) and lymphoma of the small bowel are increased in celiac disease.

3. If the gluten-free diet is used to confirm the diagnosis of nontropical sprue (celiac disease), folic acid should not be given if tropical sprue (caused by bacterial overgrowth following a bout of turista) is suspected, since the latter disorder responds to both folic acid and antibiotics.

4. Although severe mucosal atrophy of the proximal small bowel is usually caused by nontropical sprue, similar findings can be observed after a viral enteropathy, antibiotic use (neomycin), and in patients with IgA deficiency.

SUGGESTED READINGS

Auricchio S, De Ritis G, De Vincenzi, et al: Toxicity mechanisms of wheat and other cereals in celiac disease and related enteropathies. J Pediatr Gastroenterol Nutr 4:923, 1985.
Bramble MG, Zucoloto S, Wright NA, et al: Acute gluten challenge in treated adult coeliac disease: A morphometric and enzymatic study. Gut 26:169, 1985.
Koop I, Bozkurt T, Adler G, et al: Plasma cholecystokinin and pancreatic enzyme secretion in patient with coeliac sprue. Gastroenterology 25:124, 1987.
Kumar PJ: The enigma of celiac disease. Gastroenterology 89:214, 1985.
Swinson CM, Coles EC, Slavin G, et al: Coeliac disease and malignancy. Lancet 1:111, 1983.
Westergaard H: The sprue syndromes. Am J Med Sci 290(6):249, 1985.

CASE 14: SEVERE UPPER ABDOMINAL PAIN AFTER THE EVENING MEAL

A 45-year-old woman presents to the emergency room with the complaint of severe upper abdominal pain beginning 3 hours after her evening meal. The pain was first noted in the epigastrium but seems to be more severe now in the right upper quadrant. She vomited once, has no back pain or diarrhea, and is taking hydrochlorothiazide for mild hypertension. Physical examination shows normal blood pressure and temperature. Her chest and heart are unremarkable. Her bowel sounds are reduced but present. Right upper quadrant and epigastric tenderness with mild muscle guarding is noted. There is no liver or spleen enlargement. The digital rectal examination is normal. The white blood count is 12,500 with 79 segs, 15 lymphs, 4 monos and 2 eos. A serum amylase is 130 units (normal to 100 units).

BILIARY ISOTOPE CLUE

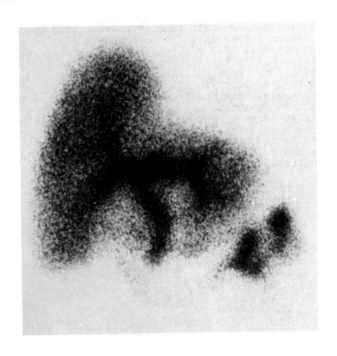

QUESTIONS (Please read the corresponding answer before proceeding to the next question.)

1. What is your differential diagnosis?

2. What additional studies would you order?

3. How would you respond to the following considerations?

   a. Nasogastric suction.

   b. Antibiotics.

   c. Analgesics.

4. What would influence your decision regarding continued medical therapy vs. early surgical intervention?

5. The patient asks you about nonsurgical measures to treat gallstones. What are they and are they appropriate for this patient?

ANSWERS

1. a. Acute cholecystitis in view of the epigastric pain
    which moved to the right upper quadrant, occurring
    several hours after a meal, with evidence of early
    muscle guarding and leukocytosis. The pain of biliary
    colic may subside for several hours and then recur in
    the right quadrant, representing the shift from
    visceral pain secondary to gallbladder obstruction to
    the somatic abdominal pain of cholecystitis.
    b. Pancreatitis should be considered since the patient
    is experiencing upper abdominal pain and tenderness and
    has a modest amylase elevation.
    c. A deeply penetrating or perforated peptic ulcer
    could give a similar picture. The amylase elevation
    may represent amylase which "leaked" into the
    peritoneal cavity.
    d. Right upper quadrant pain can also result from
    renal stones, lower lobe pneumonia or pleuritic
    disease, and parietal disorders, such as intercostal
    neuritis secondary to herpes zoster.

2. a. An obstruction series to determine if gallstones
    are visible (seen in 15% of patients with
    cholelithiasis), free air is present (absent in
    approximately 15-30% of patients with perforated
    ulcers) or signs of pancreatitis, such as sentinel
    loop, colon cut-off sign, pancreatic calcifications or
    pleural effusions. The abdominal films were
    unremarkable in this patient. The presence of a
    palpable gallbladder (not found in this patient) in an
    individual with a compatible history strongly suggests
    a diagnosis of cholecystitis. Most patients with this
    diagnosis, save for the rare case with a shrunken
    gallbladder, have distension of the gallbladder, but
    muscle guarding or "heavy" palpation may obscure the
    finding.
    b. An ultrasound of the gallbladder to evaluate for
    gallstones and pancreatitis. The examination in this
    patient revealed an edematous gallbladder which
    contained several small stones. The pancreas was not
    enlarged. The ultrasonographer reported that the
    transducer elicited discomfort when placed with gentle
    pressure over the gallbladder.
    c. Although the clinical picture was now highly
    suggestive of cholecystitis, it is conceivable that the
    gallstones were incidental findings. A biliary isotope
    scan was obtained and showed prompt filling of the
    common bile duct and duodenum, but the gallbladder did
    not fill, indicating cystic duct obstruction (see

Clue).

    d. A serum bilirubin, AST (SGOT) and ALT (SGPT) should be obtained to evaluate for ascending cholangitis and/or common bile duct obstruction. An intrahepatic gallbladder may cause sufficient perihepatitis to result in jaundice.

3. a. A nasogastric tube should be inserted during the acute phase of cholecystitis since it reduces gastric acid which can stimulate release of duodenal hormones. The procedure can also reduce the likelihood of paralytic ileus. Although this patient had bowel sounds, a nasogastric tube was inserted and attached to suction.
    b. The early phase of cholecystitis is primarily a "motor" disorder, with the gallbladder contracting against a cystic duct obstruction. Pressure builds within the wall of the gallbladder, vessels become attenuated and ischemia develops. Bacteria often gain entrance through the damaged gallbladder wall and can serve to deconjugate and reduce the bile acids, which in turn can have an irritant effect on the mucosa. The inflammatory reaction and infected bile can also result in cholangitis. Broad spectrum antibacterial coverage directed against enteric organisms should be started.
    c. Analgesics should <u>not</u> be administered until an adequate physical examination has been performed since the muscle guarding and tenderness will diminish and perhaps temporarily subside. Morphine should be avoided since it may increase the tone of the sphincter of Oddi. Demerol, 100 mg intramuscularly every 4 hours p.r.n., was ordered.

4. Early surgical intervention is required if there is evidence of an increasing inflammatory reaction, as evidenced by greater abdominal pain and/or tenderness, muscle guarding or leukocytosis. If progressive improvement is noted, as occurred in this patient, a cholecystectomy should be performed during the next several days, provided that there are no other complications that require therapy, such as cardiopulmonary disease.

5. The following nonsurgical approaches to gallstone are available:
    a. Dissolution therapy with chenodeoxycholic acid (and ursodeoxycholic acid when available) are of most benefit for radiolucent small stones which "layer" by oral cholecystography. The overall complete dissolution rate with chenodeoxycholic acid is

approximately 14% and partial dissolution in another 27% in 2 years (National Cooperative Gallstone Study) with increasing dissolution rates with prolonged therapy. Side effects of chenodeoxycholic acid include mild diarrhea and a 3% incidence of reversible hepatitis. There is a significant recurrence rate after cessation of therapy. Ursodeoxycholic acid appears more effective and safer. This patient is a good risk for surgery and was advised against dissolution therapy.

b. A lithotripsy device for sound wave fractionation of gallstones is now in clinical trials. The stones must be lucent, the gallbladder must be visualized by oral cholecystography, and very large stones (over 3 cm) do not respond well. Fragments often remain after the shock-wave therapy, requiring continued use of dissolution therapy with chenodeoxycholic and/or ursodeoxycholic acid after the procedure to complete the stone eradication and prevent re-formation. This may become an attractive alternative to surgery for selected patients, but further experience with the procedure is required.

c. Patients with symptomatic gallstone disease who are deemed unacceptable risks for surgery may be offered percutaneous catheterization of the gallbladder with installation of dissolution agents such as methyl butyl ether or monooctanoin. Although there are risks of leakage from the gallbladder and toxicity from the dissolving agents (particularly methyl butyl ether), the approach can be life-saving in selected patients.

PEARLS

1. The term "biliary colic" is not descriptive, since the pain of cystic duct obstruction is usually steady or gradually progressive without the recurrent abrupt onset and return to normal as seen in renal colic.

2. Acute cholecystitis can occur in the absence of gallstones (acalculous cholecystitis), occurring most often after trauma, unrelated surgical treatment and in critically ill patients. An early diagnosis is essential since 50% or more of such patients are found to have complications at surgery, such as gangrene, empyema or perforation of the gallbladder. The clinical features can be confusing, but ultrasonography may be helpful by demonstrating a thickened gallbladder wall, an enlarged tender gallbladder or a pericholecystic collection. At least one of these

findings was found in 90% of these patients in a recent study.

3. Choledocholithiasis occurs in approximately 15% of patients with gallstones. Mild jaundice is not uncommon in acute cholecystitis and need not necessarily represent choledocholithiasis and ascending cholangitis.

4. Palpation for an enlarged gallbladder should be performed with gentle pressure since the gallbladder may be surprisingly close to the anterior wall of the abdomen.

PITFALLS

1. Patients with gallstones may present with upper abdominal symptoms unrelated to their stone disease. Functional disorders of the stomach (nonulcer dyspepsia) or colon (irritable bowel or hepatic flexure syndrome) may be confused with biliary symptoms. Cholecystectomy in such patients often results in failure to improve or the development of new symptoms.

2. Failure to visualize the gallbladder by biliary isotope studies may be the result of thickened bile preventing access and mixing of the isotope in the gallbladder. This has been observed in patients on prolonged bowel rest, such as those treated with nasogastric suction or intravenous fluids (particularly those on prolonged total parenteral nutrition (TPN)).

3. Since the ultrasound accuracy for the detection of gallstones is approximately 97%, do not accept a "negative" ultrasound as absolute evidence for the absence of stone disease. Consider an oral cholecystogram or endoscopic retrograde cholangiopancreatogram (ERCP) if the symptoms are highly suggestive of biliary disease.

4. "Prophylactic" cholecystectomy should be avoided in asymptomatic patients with gallstones. There appears to be a long asymptomatic period (at least 2 years) between the formation of gallstones and their genesis of symptoms, as determined by a radiocarbon technique. Although surgery had been advised for asymptomatic diabetic patients with gallstones, more recent studies indicate that the surgical morbidity and mortality of these patients is not significantly different from

nondiabetic patients, perhaps due to the improved quality of postoperative care.

5. Some patients experience severe midline high epigastric pain from acute cholecystitis, which could be confused with a myocardial infarction.

SUGGESTED READINGS

Claesson BE, Holmlund DE, Matzsch TW: Microflora of the gallbladder related to duration of acute cholecystitis. Surg Gynecol Obstet 162:531, 1986.

Cope Z: Cope's Early Diagnosis of the Acute Abdomen, ed. 17. New York, Oxford University Press, 1987, pp 129-135.

Johnson LB: The importance of early diagnosis of acute acalculus cholecystitis. Surg Gynecol Obstet 164:197, 1987.

Mok HYI, Druffel ERM, Rampone WM: Chronology of cholelithiasis: Dating gallstones from atmospheric radiocarbon produced by nuclear bomb explosions. N Engl J Med 314:1075, 1986.

Ransohoff DF, Miller GL, Forsythe SB, et al: Outcome of acute cholecystitis in patients with diabetes mellitus. Ann Int Med 106:829, 1987.

Sauerbruch T, Delius M, Paumgartner G, et al: Fragmentation of gallstones by extracorporeal shock waves. N Engl J Med 318:818, 1986.

Schoenfield LJ, Lachin JM, Baum RA, et al: Chenodiol (chenodeoxycholic acid) for dissolution of gallstones: The national cooperative gallstone study. Ann Int Med 95:257, 1981.

CASE 15:   PRECAUTIONS IN MEXICO

A 55-year-old lawyer plans to take his 1st trip to Mexico
and will stay in Acapulco for 1 week. He is fearful of
developing turista and consults you regarding
recommendations for prevention or treatment. He has
generally been in good health but is taking several
aspirins daily for his low back pain.

QUESTIONS (Please read the corresponding answer before
proceeding to the next question.)

1. What are his statistical chances of developing
    diarrhea?

2. What are the most common causes of traveler's diarrhea?

3. What dietary advice would you offer?

4. Should he take prophylactic medical therapy?

5. If diarrhea occurs, what treatment should be used?

ANSWERS

1. The attack rate of traveler's diarrhea varies
    considerably, depending on the locale, but the highest
    rates occur in South America, Mexico, Africa, the
    Middle East and Asia, approaching 50% in some studies.
    Intermediate-risk regions include Southern European
    countries and several Caribbean islands. The low-risk
    destinations include the United States, Canada,
    Northern Europe, Australia, New Zealand and many
    Caribbean islands.

2. Traveler's diarrhea is not caused by traveling
    conditions or jet lag. Infectious agents are the
    primary cause and enterotoxigenic Escherichia coli is
    the most common causative agent. Less frequently
    encountered bacteria include Salmonella, Shigella, and
    Campylobacter jejuni. Enteric bacteria can be isolated
    in over 75% of the cases. Intestinal parasites such as
    amebiasis and giardiasis as well as viral enteric
    pathogens, such as rotaviruses and Norwalk-like virus,
    are occasionally found.

3. Although the better hotels in Mexico purify their
    drinking water, it is still advisable to use bottled
    water or very hot water from the hotel tap. Beer, wine
    and sodas are safe to drink. Uncooked meat, seafood
    and vegetables should be avoided, as well as unpeeled
    fruit.

4. There is evidence to support the value of large,
    frequent doses of bismuth subsalicylate (Pepto-Bismol),
    60 cc or 2 tablets, 4 times daily, as prophylaxis
    against traveler's diarrhea. Compliance may not be
    adequate and some patients develop mild tinnitus due to
    the salicylate absorption. This patient has been using
    aspirin for the back pain and should certainly avoid
    combining the agents. The risk of complications from
    the effective antibiotics (doxycycline and
    trimethoprim-sulfamethoxazole), such as skin
    photosensitivity, hemolysis or Stevens-Johnson
    syndrome, is sufficient to preclude their routine use
    for prophylaxis.

5. If several loose stools occur in an 8-hour period, the
    following program could be outlined:
    a. Although serious dehydration is uncommon, fluid
    intake should be increased but dairy products should be
    avoided.

b. Therapy with diphenoxylate (Lomotil) or loperamide (Imodium) will usually reduce the stool frequency, but should be avoided if fever or rectal bleeding occurs since invasive bacteria, such as Salmonella or Shigella, may be present. Although the improvement is somewhat slower, bismuth subsalicylate could be taken.

c. If improvement is not experienced within 24 hours, consider adding an antibiotic, such as doxycycline or trimethoprim-sulfamethoxazole. A 3-day course of antibiotic therapy is as effective as a 5-day course and reduces the likelihood of side effects.

PEARLS

1. Traveler's diarrhea usually occurs 2-3 days after the offending food or liquid has been ingested, thus the possibility that symptoms will occur <u>after</u> the patient has returned from his vacation.

2. Although the emphasis has usually been placed on water as the cause of traveler's diarrhea, food is thought to play an equal or more important role.

3. Patients at higher risk for traveler's diarrhea include those who have previously experienced a serious episode in the same country, and those who have diminished gastric acid from ulcer surgery or the use of H2-receptor antagonists. Prophylaxis with bismuth subsalicylate (or perhaps the antibiotics listed above) may be considered for such patients.

4. Traveler's diarrhea is a self-limited disorder averaging approximately 3.6 days. Therefore, affected patients intending a prolonged stay need not take any antibiotic therapy, but individuals on a brief vacation would find benefit in shortening the symptom duration.

PITFALLS

1. The photosensitivity encountered with doxycycline and trimethoprim-sulfamethoxazole would pose a particular problem for surf and sand enthusiasts in endemic areas.

2. Although most patients find complete resolution of the symptoms, some patients continue to experience crampy pain and bowel irregularity for prolonged periods of time following the eradication of the organisms. The

cause for these symptoms is unclear but undetected parasites or the development of an irritable bowel syndrome should be considered.

3. Entero-Vioform and related medications may be recommended by local physicians or pharmacists in endemic areas but should be avoided because of potential serious neurological side effects.

4. Patients advised to take bismuth subsalicylate should be advised that their tongue may become darkened and that their stools may turn black. Failure to recognize this possibility may lead patients and unwary physicians to assume that gastrointestinal bleeding has occurred.

SUGGESTED READINGS

Concensus conference. Traveler's diarrhea. JAMA 253:2700, 1985.
DuPont HL, Sullivan P, Pickering LK, et al: Symptomatic treatment of diarrhea with bismuth subsalicylate among students attending a Mexican university. Gastroenterology 73:715, 1977.
Ericsson CD, Johnson PC, Dupont HL, et al: Ciprofloxacin or trimethoprim-sulfamethoxazole as initial therapy for traveler's diarrhea. Ann Int Med 106:216, 1987.
Giannella RA: Chronic diarrhea in travelers: Diagnostic and therapeutic considerations. Rev Infect Dis 8(Suppl 2):223, 1986.
Gorbach SL: Bacterial diarrhea and its treatment. Lancet 2:1378, 1987.
Sack RB: Antimicrobial prophylaxis of traveler's diarrhea: A selected summary. Rev Infect Dis 8(Suppl 2):160, 1986.

CASE 16:   DEPRESSION AND ACUTE ODYNOPHAGIA

A 27-year-old man is brought to the emergency room by his parents who inform you that the patient had been severely depressed and may have ingested an unknown quantity of liquid drain cleaner. The patient complained of odynophagia but denied chest pain. There had been no vomiting. Physical examination showed normal vital signs. The chest and abdominal examinations were unremarkable and the stool was negative for occult blood. The CBC was normal.

CLUE

The soft palate and posterior pharynx showed hyperemia and erosions. The tongue was normal.

QUESTIONS (Please read the corresponding answer before proceeding to the next question.)

1. What would you wish to know about the liquid drain cleaner?

2. What studies would you obtain?

3. Would you insert an indwelling nasogastric tube?

4. Should antibiotics be given?

5. Is there a role for corticosteroids?

6. How should nutritional requirements be addressed?

7. What are the late complications of caustic ingestion?

ANSWERS

1. It would be helpful to have information as to whether
    this was a drain cleaner and if it is an acid or
    alkali. In this case, the substance was a commonly
    used 35% sodium hydroxide solution. Acids tend to
    produce gastric burns and may, in some cases, spare the
    esophagus.

2. a. A chest x-ray should be obtained on admission to
    determine if aspiration pneumonitis or mediastinitis is
    present. In addition, free air may be found under the
    diaphragm, indicating gastroduodenal perforation. The
    chest x-ray was negative in this patient.
    b. The finding of pharyngeal hyperemia does not
    necessarily indicate the presence of esophageal burns
    since the patient may have failed to swallow the
    liquid. Although considerable controversy has
    surrounded the question of early endoscopy, in view of
    complications experienced by those using rigid
    endoscopes or large calibre flexible instruments, the
    availability of pediatric flexible endoscopes permits
    examination of the esophagus in almost all patients.
    Although the instrument may be passed beyond areas of
    superficial esophageal erosion into the stomach,
    prudence may dictate that the identification of severe
    esophageal burns is sufficient information. If no
    pathology is identified in the esophagus or stomach,
    the patient can be discharged. The examination in this
    patient revealed severe circumferential ulceration in
    the proximal third of the esophagus and the instrument
    was not advanced into the stomach.

3. An indwelling nasogastric tube need not be used
    routinely, but some authors recommend passage of a
    string or small bore tube to maintain a lumen for
    dilatation if an esophageal stricture develops. A tube
    was not used in this patient.

4. A broad spectrum antibiotic which is effective against
    oral pharyngeal flora should be started immediately to
    reduce the likelihood of mediastinitis and sepsis.

5. The value of corticosteroids for the prevention of
    strictures after corrosive ingestion has not been
    evaluated by randomized studies (nor are such studies
    likely to be performed), thus the need to rely on
    animal experiments which suggest that this approach may
    be helpful if begun within 24-48 hours of the "burn."
    Corticosteroid therapy (usually given in large doses)

may predispose to perforation, and therefore prompts the need for concomitant antibiotic coverage. Intravenous hydrocortisone was begun in this patient and subsequently changed to oral prednisone for a period of 2 weeks.

6. Patients should be kept n.p.o. for 5-7 days, or longer, depending on the degree of mucosal damage. Dysphagia may be a problem once feedings are begun. Consider TPN, as was given in this patient, until oral feedings are well tolerated. An operative feeding jejunostomy has also been advocated.

7. The end result of corrosive ingestion may be esophageal stricture formation or fibrotic contracture of the stomach or duodenum if significant damage had occurred in these areas. A worrisome potential complication is esophageal carcinoma, which may be encountered many years after the ingestion. The risk of gastric carcinoma in patients suffering significant corrosive gastritis is uncertain.

PEARLS

1. The liquid drain cleaners affect a greater surface area of the esophagus and stomach, produce serious injury in most patients who swallow them, and are less likely to be vomited back than the older granular products which are said to have produced serious injury in less than 25% of patients.

2. The most commonly used system to classify corrosive burns is as follows:
   a. 1st degree: mucosal hyperemia, edema and superficial sloughing.
   b. 2nd degree: deeper tissue damage, transmucosal involvement with exudate, ulceration, erosions and loss of mucosa.
   c. 3rd degree: erosion through the esophagus into the mediastinal, pleural or peritoneal cavities.

3. The effect of acids on the stomach is enhanced by the accompanying pylorospasm which causes the acid to pool in the antrum, where maximal damage occurs.

4. If endoscopy is prohibited by the severity of the esophageal burns, consider a water-soluble upper gastrointestinal contrast study if there is concern about the severity of gastroduodenal involvement.

Known or suspected perforation is a contraindication to endoscopy since insufflation of air (necessary for visualization) may cause greater leakage of gas and acid into the peritoneal cavity.

PITFALLS

1. Although vinegar or other weak acids had been advocated for the purpose of neutralizing alkalis, the damage has already been done (it occurs within seconds) and the weak acid may itself serve as an additional irritant.

2. Failure to recognize that hoarseness or laryngeal stridor often represents aspiration of the corrosive could delay appropriate therapy. Such patients may require intubation. Careful attention must be directed toward the airway.

3. Do not delay esophageal dilatations if a stricture becomes apparent. The dilatations are usually begun by the 2nd or 3rd week. A longer delay allows the fibrosis to contract further and makes dilatations more difficult. There is always a risk of perforation during the procedure.

4. Patients may have misleadingly few symptoms after acid ingestion, but the antral duodenal disease may progress to outlet obstruction.

SUGGESTED READINGS

Cello JP, Fogel RP, Boland R: Liquid caustic ingestion. Arch Intern Med 140:501, 1980.
Dilawari JB, Singh S, Rao PN, et al: Corrosive acid ingestion in man--a clinical and endoscopic study.   Gut 25:183, 1984.
Goldman LP, Weigert JM: Corrosive substance ingestion: A review. Am J Gastroenterol 79:85, 1984.
Zamir O, Lernau OZ, Mogle P, et al: Corrosive injury to the stomach due to acid ingestion. Am Surg 51:170, 1985.

CASE 17: ABDOMINAL PAIN, FEVER, DIARRHEA AND A LEG RASH

A 26-year-old nurse complains of postprandial crampy pain and intermittent diarrhea beginning 2 months prior to her visit to your office. Fever to approximately 100 F was noted in the previous week, associated with a tender rash on both legs. There has been no rectal bleeding. She describes a several pound weight loss. Her only medication has been loperamide for diarrhea. Her family history was unremarkable. Physical examination shows normal vital signs. Bowel sounds are normal. Her abdomen is soft but there is "fullness" and some tenderness in the right lower quadrant. The rectal examination is normal and the stool is negative for occult blood. Bilateral erythematous nodules are found on both legs. The hemoglobin is 12.5 g%, white blood count 11,400 with 78 segs, 18 lymphs, 3 monos and 1 eosin.

SMALL BOWEL BARIUM CLUE

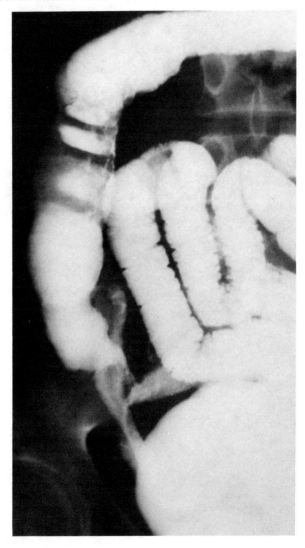

QUESTIONS (Please read the corresponding answer before proceeding to the next question.)

1. What diagnoses would you consider?

2. What would be the most direct diagnostic approach?

3. What is the bilateral leg rash?

4. What treatment would you offer?

5. How long would you continue the medical therapy?

6. What is the likelihood that this patient will require surgery and for what complication?

ANSWERS

1. a. A young woman with diarrhea of several months
    duration, low grade fever and right lower quadrant
    tenderness should suggest the possibility of Crohn's
    disease, either ileitis or ileocolitis.
    b. Although rare, chronic appendicitis could recur
    intermittently for several months and subsequently
    result in an appendiceal abscess. Tuberculosis of the
    ileocecal region could also present with similar
    symptoms, but this disease is also rare in this
    country.
    c. Right lower quadrant pain and tenderness in a young
    woman should raise the possibility of pelvic
    inflammatory disease, perhaps a tubo-ovarian abscess,
    although the chronic course and history of diarrhea
    would be atypical.

2. Since the abdominal examination shows no evidence of
    bowel obstruction (normal bowel sounds, no distension,
    no vomiting) an obstruction series is not likely to be
    helpful. An ultrasound of the right lower quadrant
    could provide information regarding a possible abscess
    but it was not performed in this case. If appendicitis
    was a strong consideration, a barium enema would have
    been performed, but the clinical picture was
    sufficiently compelling for Crohn's disease that the
    initial study was an upper gastrointestinal barium
    study with small bowel follow-through. It showed edema
    and ulcerations in the distal 10 cm of the terminal
    ileum and contraction of the cecum, without evidence of
    fistula or obstruction (see Clue). There was no
    suggestion of an abscess.

3. Erythema nodosum is the most common cutaneous lesion in
    Crohn's disease, occurring in approximately 15% of
    patients. Although the lesions, which usually appear
    on the anterior surface of the lower extremities, tend
    to correlate with the activity of the bowel disease,
    they may appear prior to an exacerbation. Improvement
    generally occurs when the bowel disease is medically
    (or surgically) brought under control. The healed
    lesions can be identified by the persisting
    pigmentation. Pyoderma gangrenosum is less common but
    more debilitating. The disorder begins as one or more
    erythematous papules or vesicles which subsequently
    develop into ulcerating lesions with undermined, ragged
    edges. The disease usually responds to medical or
    surgical management of the Crohn's disorder, but

medically unresponsive cases as well as those which
recur after surgery have been reported.

4. This patient had signs and symptoms of acute
   inflammation of the terminal ileum. The National
   Cooperative Crohn's disease study indicates that
   sulfasalazine appears to be less effective for Crohn's
   disease of the small bowel than for ulcerative or
   Crohn's colitis. This patient was started on oral
   prednisone, 60 mg daily. Her pain began to improve
   after several days and the tenderness and "mass"
   (inflamed and edematous terminal ileum) in the right
   lower quadrant also diminished. The erythema nodosum
   responded dramatically. Her diet was gradually
   increased and the prednisone dose was reduced.

5. Ideally, the prednisone should be gradually tapered
   over several weeks or months and eventually
   discontinued. Unfortunately, many patients, such as
   this young woman, develop recurrent symptoms when the
   dose is reduced below 10 or 15 mg/day, thus requiring
   long-term maintenance therapy.

6. Approximately 85% of patients with Crohn's disease
   require a major surgical procedure. Small bowel
   obstruction, fistulas and abscess, in that order, are
   the most common causes in ileitis. The most common
   indication in Crohn's colitis is intractability. The
   recurrence rate after resection and reanastamosis is
   approximately 50% in 10 years, with the recurrence
   generally occurring immediately proximal to the suture
   line.

PEARLS

1. Since prednisone is largely bound to albumin, it is the
   unbound fraction which has biologic activity.
   Therefore, patients with a low serum albumin will have
   a greater steroid effect (and complications) at any
   given dose than patients with a normal serum albumin.

2. Crohn's disease (or ulcerative colitis) occurring in
   the prepubertal years may stunt linear growth,
   indicating the need for aggressive medical or surgical
   therapy. The growth retardation may be due to
   inadequate caloric intake rather than the direct effect
   of the inflammatory bowel disease.

3. The corticosteroid side effects can be diminished somewhat if the medication is given on an every other day basis, but this should not be done during the acute phase of the disease.

4. The perineal complications of Crohn's disease (fistula and abscess) occur more frequently in patients with left-sided colitis. These lesions tend to respond to oral metronidazole, but the Antabuse effect and peripheral neuropathy associated with this drug require careful observation.

5. An elevation of the alkaline phosphatase in patients with Crohn's disease usually indicates fat infiltration of the liver or pericholangitis. Gallstones occur more frequently in patients with ileitis, usually secondary to a diminished bile acid pool. Sclerosing cholangitis is more common in ulcerative colitis than Crohn's disease.

PITFALLS

1. If a patient is operated on because of right lower quadrant pain and tenderness which suggests appendicitis, a resection of the ileum should not be performed if terminal ileitis is found. Approximately 30% of such patients will improve spontaneously with no recurrence of their ileitis. If the cecum is grossly uninvolved, an appendectomy should be performed to reduce the confusion should similar symptoms recur.

2. A right-sided hydronephrosis is occasionally overlooked in patients with acute inflammatory disease of the terminal ileum which can result in compression of the right ureter. The process can be detected easily by renal ultrasound. Improvement usually occurs if the ileitis resolves with appropriate therapy, but the retroperitoneal fibrosis which may occur with chronic ileitis can result in permanent hydronephrosis. Renal calculi occur in approximately 15% of patients with inflammatory bowel disease, possibly due to chronic dehydration and increased oxalate absorption.

3. If surgery for obstruction or fistula is required, the goal should be removal of only the grossly involved gut. Patients with multiple short strictures can sometimes be managed by "mini-resections" of the strictured areas.

4. Patients with symptomatic hemorrhoids associated with diarrhea should have appropriate studies to rule out Crohn's disease before any consideration for hemorrhoidectomy. Failure to recognize the presence of Crohn's disease can lead to nonhealing of the hemorrhoidectomy wounds, resulting in considerable pain and disability.

5. If pregnancy is a planned event, it is advisable to avoid conception during periods of active inflammatory bowel disease since spontaneous abortion may be increased. Approximately 50% of women have no change in their symptoms if pregnancy occurs during a period of absolute or relative remission, 25% seem to improve somewhat, and 25% become worse. We have encountered 2 patients who perforated their terminal ileum just immediately prior to labor, 1 of whom was induced with pitressin and subsequently had a pelvic abscess drained and the other had an emergency resection and ileostomy followed by a cesarean section.

SUGGESTED READINGS

Farmer RG, Whelan G, Fazio VW: Long-term follow-up of patients with Crohn's disease: Relationship between the clinical pattern and prognosis. Gastroenterology 88:1818, 1985.

Jakobovits J, Schuster MM: Metronidazole therapy for Crohn's disease and associated fistulae. Am J Gastroenterol 79:533, 1984.

James SP, Strober W, Quinn TC, et al: Crohn's disease: New concepts of pathogenesis and current approaches to treatment. Dig Dis Sci 32:1297, 1987.

Kelts DG, Grand RJ, Shen G, et al: Nutritional basis of growth failure in children and adolescents with Crohn's disease. Gastroenterology 76:720, 1979.

Prantera C, Levenstein S, Capocaccia R, et al: Prediction of surgery for obstruction in Crohn's ileitis. Dig Dis Sci 32:1363, 1987.

Sorensen VZ, Olsen BG, Binder V: Life prospects and quality of life in patients with Crohn's disease. Gut 28:382, 1987.

Summers RW, Switz DM, Sessions JT Jr, et al: National Cooperative Crohn's Disease Study: Results of drug treatment. Gastroenterology 77:847, 1979.

CASE 18:   ALCOHOL AND JAUNDICE

A 39-year-old male presents to the emergency room with the complaint of nausea, vomiting and upper abdominal pain. He has a 10-year history of approximately 150 g of daily alcohol use, and weight loss of 25 pounds in the past several months. There has been no drug use and the patient was not under medical care. Physical examination showed evidence of mild muscle wasting. He was icteric, had several spider nevi on the upper chest, and palmer erythema. The abdomen showed tenderness in the right upper quadrant. The liver measured 15 cm from the superior to the inferior margin, the spleen was not palpable and there was no evidence of ascites. The hemoglobin was 10.6 g% with macrocytic indices, the bilirubin was 5.8 mg%, the alkaline phosphatase was 230 units (normal to 85 units), the serum ALT (SGPT) was 64 units and the AST (SGOT) was 190 units. The amylase was 130 units (normal to 100 units). The serum albumin was 3.2 g%.

LIVER BIOPSY CLUE

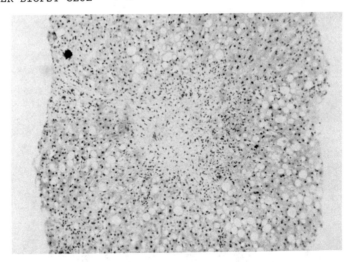

QUESTIONS (Please read the corresponding answer before proceeding to the next question.)

1. What is your differential diagnosis?

2. What additional laboratory or imaging studies would you order?

3. In view of the alcohol history, what is the value of performing a liver biopsy?

4. What are the histologic features of alcoholic hepatitis?

5. What nutritional program would you outline?

6. How does alcohol lead to hepatocellular damage?

ANSWERS

1. a. Alcoholic liver disease is likely. Note that the SGOT/SGPT ratio exceeds 2:1, a finding which is highly suggestive of this diagnosis.
   b. Alcoholic pancreatitis is associated with compression of the common bile duct, thus leading to cholestatic features, in as many as 10% of patients.
   c. Acute cholecystitis.
   d. Acute nonalcoholic liver disease.

2. a. Ultrasound of the liver, gallbladder and pancreas. This showed a homogeneous enlargement of the liver. The gallbladder was normal and the bile ducts were not enlarged. The pancreas appeared normal.
   b. Coagulation studies. The prothrombin time was 2.9" over control. The partial thromboplastin time (PTT) and platelet count were normal.
   c. Viral serologic studies were normal.

3. Approximately 20% of patients with clinical features compatible with alcoholic liver disease have a nonalcoholic process, thus the need to perform a liver biopsy in all such patients. It would be unfortunate to overlook the presence of such disorders as granulomatous or chronic active hepatitis, which may be treatable. In addition, the finding of alcoholic hepatitis in the presence of cirrhosis significantly increases the 1 and 5 year mortality rate when compared with alcoholic cirrhotics without hepatitis.

4. a. Fat deposition, a nonspecific finding occurring in approximately 80% of patients by the time of liver biopsy.
   b. Mallory bodies (alcoholic hyaline), often centrolobular and present in approximately 50% of patients.
   c. Varying degrees of neutrophilic inflammatory reaction.
   d. Perivenular sclerosis (a rim of fibrous tissue around the central veins) appears to be a marker indicating a greater likelihood of progression to cirrhosis, since the process tends to extend toward the portal space. There is no obvious correlation between the fat content of the liver and the degree of perivenular sclerosis.

This patient had evidence of perivenular sclerosis, fatty infiltration, and neutrophilic inflammation (see Clue).

5. The anorexia and nausea precluded adequate oral protein supplementation. Several days of peripheral alimentation were begun, but the patient's oral intake did not improve and he was changed to total parenteral nutrition (TPN). Branched chain amino acids were not given in view of the added cost and the failure of controlled studies to show any clear advantage in these patients. There was no evidence of hepatic encephalopathy. The patient was able to tolerate increasing high protein oral feedings after 10 days of TPN.

6. The liver plays a major role in removing alcohol from the blood. Approximately 80% of the ethanol entering the liver is oxidized to acetaldehyde which is subsequently oxidized to acetate. Patients with alcoholic liver disease have reduced hepatocyte cytosolic acetaldehyde dehydrogenase levels which lead to higher cellular acetaldehyde after ethanol ingestion. The accumulating acetaldhyde appears to have a damaging effect on mitochondria and thus result in hepatocyte necrosis. Nonalcoholic liver disease can also lead to a similar decrease in the patient's ability to metabolize alcohol, thus providing a rationale for such individuals to abstain from alcohol ingestion. Additional factors relating alcohol to hepatocellular damage include the formation of free radicals during ethanol metabolism, immunologic factors and changes in permeability of the hepatocyte membrane.

PEARLS

1. Women are more prone to develop alcoholic cirrhosis than men. At any given daily alcoholic intake, a higher percentage of women will develop cirrhosis and tend to do so with a shorter drinking history.

2. Patients with alcoholic hepatitis can present with spider nevi and palmar erythema, as well as esophageal varices, so that these criteria cannot be used to distinguish hepatitis from cirrhosis.

3. Alcoholic hepatitis should be viewed as a potentially reversible disorder. Such patients with cirrhosis and

portal hypertension may also show a significant decrease in portal pressure if alcohol intake ceases and nutrition improves.

4. There is very little evidence to support the value of corticosteroid therapy for acute alcoholic hepatitis. It is best to avoid this approach since these patients are particularly prone to infectious complications as well as the other side effects associated with corticosteroids.

5. A 4 oz glass of wine and a bottle of beer each contain approximately 12 g of alcohol, while 1 oz of whisky contains approximately 10 g. It is unusual for patients drinking less than 60 g of alcohol daily to develop chronic alcoholic liver disease.

PITFALLS

1. It is prudent to entertain a degree of skepticism regarding a patient's claims to have "given up drinking" several weeks prior to his presentation with symptoms of alcoholic hepatitis. Cessation of alcohol ingestion in such patients is either a result of their recognition of the dangers of drinking or, more likely, that they were too sick to drink.

2. Anorexia and nausea are dominant symptoms in acute alcoholic hepatitis and do not subside because the patient has been hospitalized. Consider nutritional strategies on admission and do not avoid protein intake for fear of hepatic encephalopathy. The risks of amino acids given by peripheral parenteral nutrition (PPN) or TPN can be minimized by careful observation.

3. Some patients with alcoholic hepatitis present with predominantly cholestatic biochemical features, with significant jaundice, very high alkaline phosphatase and only mildly elevated SGOT and SGPT. These features could lead to an erroneous diagnosis of common bile duct obstruction from gallstone disease or pancreatic compression. Failure to show a dilated common bile duct by ultrasound should clarify the issue.

4. Although chronic alcohol use can increase the activity of the cytochrome oxidase system in the smooth endoplasmic reticulum, thus enhancing drug

detoxification and making sedation more difficult, the severely intoxicated patient may be overly sensitive to sedatives and narcotics.

5. There is considerable pessimism about the ability of alcoholics to follow an alcohol withdrawal process. Nevertheless, no patient should be discharged from hospital without an effort made to enter the patient in AA or some other program.

SUGGESTED READINGS

Achord JL: Malnutrition and the role of nutritional support in alcoholic liver disease. Am J Gastroenterol 82:1, 1987.

Cohen JA, Kaplan MM: The SGOT/SGPT ratio--an indicator of alcoholic liver disease. Dig Dis Sci 24:835, 1979.

Matthewson K, Mardini H Al, Bartlett K, et al: Impaired acetaldehyde metabolism in patients with non-alcoholic liver disorders. Gut 27:756, 1986.

Mendenhall CL, Anderson S, Garcia-Pont P, et al: Short-term and long-term survival in patients with alcoholic hepatitis treated with oxandrolone and prednisolone. N Engl J Med 311:1464, 1984.

Orrego H, Blake JE, Blendis M, et al: Prognosis of alcoholic cirrhosis in the presence and absence of alcoholic hepatitis. Gastroenterology 92:208, 1987.

Worner TM, Lieber CS: Perivenular fibrosis as precursor lesion of cirrhosis. JAMA 254:627, 1985.

CASE 19: LIVER FUNCTION DISTURBANCE IN A YOUNG WOMAN

A 28-year-old real estate agent presented to her local
physician with the history of fatigue, anorexia, low grade
fevers, intermittent mild right upper quadrant discomfort
and arthralgias for approximately 6 months. Her only
medication is aspirin for her joint symptoms. Her past
medical history is unremarkable. She denied drug or
alcohol use. Physical examination showed no organ
enlargement or abdominal tenderness. A biochemical profile
revealed the following: AST (SGOT) 180 units (normal to
40 units), ALT (SGPT) 115 units (normal to 40 units),
albumin 4.2 g%, bilirubin 1.0 mg%, and alkaline phosphatase
125 units (normal to 85 units). The CBC was normal.
Additional studies were ordered and showed the HBsAg,
HBsAb and HBcAb to be normal.

LIVER BIOPSY CLUE

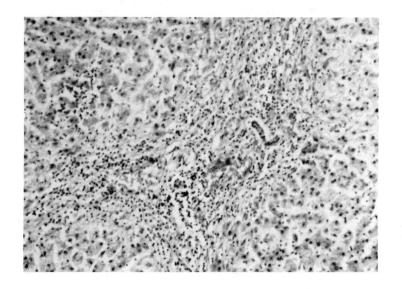

QUESTIONS (Please read the corresponding answer before proceeding to the next question.)

1. What diagnoses would you consider?

2. What additional noninvasive studies would be helpful?

3. What diagnostic study is now likely to establish the diagnosis?

4. Outline a plan of therapy.

5. How long would you continue the program?

ANSWERS

1. a. There is biochemical evidence of hepatitis. The
   history of symptoms for 6 months suggests a "chronic"
   category, while the arthralgias would implicate an
   immunologic disorder, such as chronic active hepatitis.
   b. Considerable aspirin use, as for rheumatoid
   arthritis, can cause a nonspecific hepatitis which
   resolves with cessation of therapy. Closer questioning
   in this patient revealed an intermittent daily use of
   4-6 aspirins, a dose unlikely to produce signs of
   hepatitis.
   c. Idiopathic hepatitis in someone under age 35 should
   raise the possibility of metabolic disorders, such as
   Wilson's disease, alpha-1 antitrypsin deficiency and
   iron storage disease.
   d. Infectious mononucleosis.

2. a. Serum protein electrophoresis. It showed a gamma
   globulin of 2.1 g%, suggesting an autoimmune disorder.
   b. In an effort to rule out Wilson's disease, the
   serum copper and ceruloplasmin levels, as well as a
   slitlamp examination for Kayser-Fleischer rings, were
   performed, all of which were normal. The serum iron
   and iron binding capacity and the alpha-1 antitrypsin
   levels were normal. There was no serologic evidence of
   Epstein-Barr disease.
   c. An ultrasound study of the liver to evaluate
   parenchymal and biliary status was unremarkable.

3. A liver biopsy would provide the most useful
   information regarding the nature of the liver disorder
   and for determining the course of therapy. The
   histology showed a periportal inflammatory reaction
   with evidence of piecemeal necrosis (inflammation
   extending beyond the limiting plate and engulfing
   surrounding hepatocytes). In addition, there was
   evidence of bridging necrosis, since the inflammation
   tended to extend from one portal space to another (see
   Clue). This is consistent with a diagnosis of chronic
   active hepatitis. The parenchymal copper and iron
   content were normal.

4. A course of prednisone therapy should be initiated. A
   daily dose of 40-60 mg is usually tapered to a
   maintenance dose of 15-20 mg. Although the results are
   not improved, the addition of an immunosuppressive
   agent, such as azathioprine, may permit a reduction in
   the daily prednisone dosage, but the potential side
   effects, such as marrow suppression, should also be

considered.   Azathioprine is not effective as single
drug therapy.

5. Biochemical and clinical improvement often occur more
rapidly than the histologic response. A repeat liver
biopsy should be obtained after 1 year of therapy.

PEARLS

1. The drugs most often associated with chronic active
hepatitis (CAH) are methyldopa and nitrofurantoin.
Other drugs implicated in the etiology of CAH include
isoniazid, sulfonamides, phenylbutazone and gold.

2. Bridging necrosis between neighboring portal areas is
probably the forerunner of fibrosis and cirrhosis and
should prompt corticosteroid therapy. Piecemeal
necrosis with only minimal elevation of the
transaminase (less than twice normal) and with no
significant gamma globulin elevation need not
necessarily be treated with corticosteroids but should
be followed clinically and biochemically, with a repeat
liver biopsy in approximately 1 year if there is no
spontaneous resolution.

3. Wilson's disease should be considered in all patients
younger than 35 and in all patients with HBsAg negative
CAH since this is a treatable disease. Alpha-1
antitrypsin deficiency in adults is usually associated
with pulmonary and liver disease. Liver biopsy shows
characteristic PAS positive globules in the
hepatocytes.

4. The presence of cirrhosis as well as CAH is not a
contraindication to corticosteroid therapy, but a
favorable response is less likely. Patients with CAH
and a positive HBsAg do not respond to corticosteroid
therapy.

PITFALLS

1. Transaminase elevations over 500 units are often
considered evidence of acute viral hepatitis but
similar biochemical findings have been encountered in
15% of patients with CAH, who usually have severe liver
disease. Failure to recognize the presence of "acute"

chronic active hepatitis may result in the withholding of corticosteroid therapy which could be highly beneficial for such patients.

2. If there is no clinical or biochemical evidence of improvement after approximately 1 year of corticosteroid therapy, the treatment should be stopped. The risks of side effects probably outweigh the potential benefits of treatment at that point.

3. About 1/2 the patients who respond to therapy will relapse when corticosteroids are discontinued. Cessation of therapy should not be attempted until the liver biopsy shows either normal histology or chronic persistent hepatitis. Patients who relapse usually respond to the same initial treatment program but will probably require long-term maintenance therapy.

4. Failure to obtain an adequate liver biopsy core, as evidenced by the inability to demonstrate at least 2 portal spaces, may lead to an incorrect diagnosis.

SUGGESTED READINGS

Czaja AJ, Wolf AM, Baggenstss AH: Laboratory assessment of severe chronic active liver disease during and after corticosteroid therapy: Correlation of serum transaminase and gamma globulin levels with histologic features. Gastroenterology 80:687, 1981.
Davis GL, Czaja AJ, Ludwig J: Development and prognosis of histologic cirrhosis in corticosteroid-treated hepatitis B surface antigen-negative chronic active hepatitis. Gastroenterology 87:1222, 1984.
Gitlin N: Corticosteroid therapy for chronic active hepatitis. Am J Gastroenterol 79:573, 1984.
Hazzi C: Diagnosis and management of chronic active hepatitis. Am J Gastroenterol 81:85, 1986.
Maddrey WC: Subdivisions of idiopathic autoimmune chronic active hepatitis. Hepatology 7:1372, 1985.
Vento S, Nouri-Aria KT, Eddleston AL: Immune mechanisms in autoimmune chronic active hepatitis. Scand J Gastroenterol (Suppl) 114:91, 1985.

CASE 20: ALCOHOLISM, LIVER DYSFUNCTION AND CONFUSION

A 41-year-old woman has been diagnosed as having alcoholic cirrhosis by liver biopsy 2 years prior to admission. She has received outpatient diuretic therapy for mild to moderate ascites. Her alcohol ingestion has diminished although some heavier weekend drinking continues. She takes an occasional tranquilizer but denies narcotic use. Increasing fatigue and confusion was noted by her family and prompted admission to the emergency room. Physical examination reveals a cachectic patient who is somewhat confused as to place, person and time. She is slightly icteric. Her abdomen is mildly distended with a suggestion of shifting dullness. The liver measures 12 cm and the spleen is not palpable. There is no peripheral edema. Asterixis can be demonstrated and her deep tendon reflexes are somewhat hyperactive. The hemoglobin is 10.3 g%, white blood count 3,800, bilirubin 3.5 mg%, albumin 2.8 g%, AST (SGOT) 78 units, and prothrombin time 3.3 seconds over control.

EEG CLUE

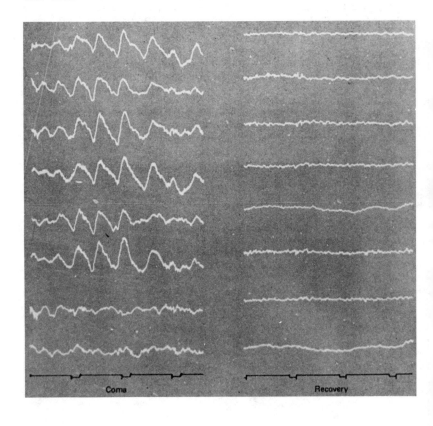

QUESTIONS (Please read the corresponding answer before proceeding to the next question.)

1. If you are considering hepatic encephalopathy as a possibility, how could you substantiate the diagnosis?

2. What factors could precipitate hepatic encephalopathy in this patient?

3. Outline three different theories for the etiology of hepatic encephalopathy.

4. What is the role for the following therapeutic agents in this patient?

   a. Lactulose.

   b. Neomycin.

   c. Intravenous branched chain amino acids.

   d. Corticosteroids.

   e. Total parenteral nutrition.

ANSWERS

1. a. The presence of asterixis should suggest hepatic
        encephalopathy, but this finding can be observed in
        other forms of metabolic encephalopathy.
    b. An arterial or venous ammonia level could be
        obtained. Although ammonia is believed to play an
        important role in the genesis of hepatic
        encephalopathy, the blood ammonia levels are not
        sufficiently predictive to be routinely used for the
        diagnosis of hepatic encephalopathy. Ammonia combines
        with alpha-ketoglutaric acid to form glutamine, which
        has been reported to be elevated in the spinal fluid of
        patients with hepatic encephalopathy, although this
        measurement has not become a routine clinical approach.
    c. An EEG was obtained in this patient and showed
        evidence of slow waves (delta waves), having a
        frequency of 2-4 cycles/second (Clue shows slow waves
        on left side and normal waves on right). This
        pattern, however, may be observed in patients with
        other forms of encephalopathy resulting from pulmonary,
        renal or congestive failure.
    d. The diagnosis of hepatic encephalopathy is
        established by clinical rather than laboratory
        criteria.

2. Her hepatic encephalopathy may have resulted from:
    a. Superimposed alcoholic hepatitis, thus
        decompensating her chronic liver disease.
    b. Aggressive diuretic therapy may have resulted in
        dehydration which led to azotemia and hyperammonemia.
        The BUN and creatinine, however, were normal.
    c. GI bleeding may lead to hypotension with subsequent
        decreased hepatic, renal and cerebral perfusion.
        Although the patient was anemic, there were no other
        features to support this possibility.
    d. The mental changes may have been the result of
        tranquilizer use and this might NOT be hepatic
        encephalopathy. Asterixis, however, would be unlikely
        in that setting.
    e. Other potential causes include sepsis, excess
        protein intake leading to "meat" intoxication, heart
        failure and electrolyte abnormalities,

3. a. Ammonia: Excess ammonia production causes cerebral
        neurotoxicity.
    b. Synergistic neurotoxins: Ammonia, mercaptans and
        fatty acids accumulate in the brain.

c. False neurotransmitters: The accumulation of octopamine and phenylethanolamine displace dopamine and norepinephrine and result in neural inhibition.

4. a. Lactulose is neither hydrolyzed nor absorbed from the gut and is metabolized by colonic flora to short-chain fatty acids which lower the colonic pH and and favors the conversion of NH3 to NH4, which is trapped in the gut. Lactulose was given to this patient.
    b. Neomycin works by decreasing the concentration of urease-containing bacteria in the colonic flora, thus decreasing the production of ammonia from proteins and amino acids. Small amounts of the antibiotic can be absorbed and can rarely lead to nephrotoxicity or ototoxicity, particularly in the presence of azotemia.
    c. Aromatic amino acids appear to increase in hepatic encephalopathy while branched chain amino acids decrease. The change in this ratio has been felt to contribute to the disorder, but intravenous branched chain amino acids are expensive and their benefit is controversial. This therapy was not used in this patient.
    d. Although corticosteroids are frequently used when other treatments fail, the experience with hepatic encephalopathy has not been impressive and there is little enthusiasm for this therapy.
    e. The administration of amino acids and albumin may lead to increased ammonia production. Although not indicated during acute hepatic encephalopathy (also consider the risk of the central venous pressure (CVP) in a patient with a coagulopathy), cautious administration to malnourished patients incapable of taking oral feedings should be considered once the encephalopathic features resolve.

PEARLS

1. A low protein diet, 30-60 g/day in divided amounts, is required for patients demonstrating intermittent signs of hepatic encephalopathy. Vegetable protein appears to be better tolerated than animal protein from the standpoint of cerebral function, possibly due to its lesser tendency to generate ammonia in the gut and to the associated intake of fiber which aids in the elimination of ammonia.

2. The psychomotor disturbances of chronic hepatic
    encephalopathy are not the result of demonstrable
    organic cerebral pathology. If liver dysfunction is
    sufficiently severe as to preclude outpatient
    management of chronic hepatic encephalopathy, the
    possibility of liver transplantation should be
    considered. Transplant teams are reluctant to operate
    on alcoholic patients unless a convincing duration of
    sobriety can be demonstrated. Transplantation has also
    been performed successfully in patients suffering from
    acute fulminant viral hepatitis.

3. Although lactulose depends upon colonic bacteria for
    its action, it surprisingly appears to work
    synergistically with neomycin, which significantly
    reduces the bacterial population.

4. Although patients with acute hepatic encephalopathy are
    usually jaundiced, patients with cirrhosis (and
    particularly those who have undergone a portal-systemic
    shunt) may demonstrate intermittent psychomotor changes
    without evidence of jaundice or other deterioration of
    their liver function tests.

PITFALLS

1. Lactulose can produce sufficient diarrhea to result in
    hypokalemia, dehydration, serum sodium over
    145 mg/liter and alkalosis. The azotemia is unwanted
    in these patients since it raises the blood ammonia
    level, as does hypokalemia. These side effects are
    more likely to occur when the daily dose exceeds
    100 ml. Other side effects include gaseousness and
    crampy abdominal discomfort.

2. Patients with alcoholic liver disease may fall and
    sustain a subdural hematoma, which could be
    misdiagnosed as hepatic encephalopathy. Consider the
    possibility and obtain a CT scan of the brain when
    appropriate.

3. Patients with liver disease are often sensitive to
    sedatives and narcotics. The prolonged somnolence or
    sleep induced by these agents could be misdiagnosed as
    hepatic encephalopathy.

4. Blood drawn for a venous ammonia level should be taken
    with care. Flexing of the fist or prolonged use of a
    tourniquet can release sufficient ammonia from the

muscles to significantly elevate the blood level. Blood should preferably be drawn from a large vein without the use of a tourniquet. If the latter is required, it should be released after the needle insertion and the needle allowed to stay in the vein for several minutes before the venesection is performed.

SUGGESTED READINGS

Branch RA: Is there increased cerebral sensitivity to benzodiazepines in chronic liver disease? Hepatology 7:773, 1987.
Butterworth RF, Giguere JF, Michaud J, et al: Ammonia: Key factor in the pathogenesis of hepatic encephalopathy. Neurochem Pathol 6:1, 1987.
Fraser CL, Arieff AI: Hepatic encephalopathy. N Engl J Med 313:865, 1985.
Gitlin N: Subclinical portal-systemic encephalopathy. Am J Gastroenterol 83:8, 1988.
Sherlock S: Chronic portal systemic encephalopathy: Update 1987. Gut 28:1043, 1987.
Silk DBA: Branched chain amino acids in liver disease: Fact or fantasy? Gut 27:S1,103, 1986.

CASE 21: CHRONIC RIGHT UPPER QUADRANT "BURNING" PAIN

A 63-year-old woman has a 15-year history of diabetes controlled with oral hypoglycemic therapy. She is referred to your outpatient clinic with the history of continuous "burning" right upper quadrant pain and tenderness for 3 months. Numerous studies have been obtained by her local physician, including an upper GI barium x-ray, ultrasound of the liver and pancreas, barium enema and CT scan of the upper abdomen. An upper GI endoscopy was negative. Routine biochemical studies have shown a fluctuating blood sugar and an alkaline phosphatase of 120 units (normal to 85 units) but have otherwise been unremarkable. Viral serologic studies were negative.

CLUE

Tenderness in the right upper quadrant did not change when the rectus muscle was tensed.

QUESTIONS

1. What clinical features make gallbladder disease unlikely?

2. What findings on physical examination could distinguish parietal from visceral pain?

3. What dermatome innervates the umbilicus?

4. What is the most likely explanation for the pain in this patient?

5. List several other possibilities for parietal pain of this nature.

ANSWERS

1. Gallstone disease is an unlikely explanation for
    chronic continuous pain. The inflammatory reaction
    would have led to signs of peritonitis or would have
    been reflected in the white blood count. The mild
    elevation of alkaline phosphatase is not unusual in
    diabetics, often representing fatty infiltration.
    The normal CT scan would reduce the likelihood of
    pancreatic carcinoma and liver metastasis. There could
    be concern about the right kidney, but, again, the CT
    scan and ultrasound study showed no evidence of
    hydronephrosis.

2. Right upper quadrant tenderness could represent
    parietal or visceral pathology. The tenderness was
    located on the right costal margin and upper quadrant.
    When the rectus muscle is tensed by having the patient
    perform a 45-degree sit-up, tenderness from visceral
    causes usually diminishes (the rectus serves as a
    "splint"), while parietal tenderness is unchanged or
    even more severe. This patient showed no lessening of
    the tenderness with rectus tensing. Pinching of the
    skin (appropriately termed the "pinch test")
    bilaterally in upper and lower quadrants can also be
    used to detect parietal pain. (It was positive in the
    right upper quadrant of this patient.)

3. T8 and T9 innervate the lower costal area and upper
    quadrants of the abdomen. T10 innervates the
    umbilicus.

4. This patient probably has a diabetic thoracoabdominal
    neuropathy in the T8-T9 dermatomes. The pain usually
    begins in the 5th or 6th decade and is often described
    as "burning," and very sensitive to touch. Paraspinal
    and abdominal muscle EMG may show denervation changes
    (not performed in this patient).

5. a. Herpes zoster may present with severe radicular
    pain prior to the appearance of the characteristic
    vesicles. Postherpetic neuralgia may continue for many
    months after the dermatitis subsides.
    b. Intercostal neuritis secondary to nerve compression
    from spinal disease.
    c. Although this patient had no previous abdominal
    surgery, consider the possibility of incisional
    neuritis when appropriate.

d. The slipping rib syndrome can produce costal margin
and upper abdominal discomfort. It appears to be
caused by abnormal mobility of the anterior
interchondral articulations of the 8th, 9th and 10th
ribs, leading to nerve compression. The diagnosis can
be established by the "hooking maneuver," accomplished
by hooking the examiner's fingers under the costal
margin and pulling anteriorly, reproducing (or
exceeding) the typical pain.

PEARLS

1. Diabetic thoracoabdominal neuropathy often occurs in
conjunction with other neuropathies, such as peripheral
neuropathy, autonomic neuropathy of the
gastrointestinal tract or diabetic neuroretinopathy.
The pain tends to subside spontaneously within 6-20
months. The pain and frustration engendered by this
disorder may respond to tricyclic antidepressant
therapy.

2. An acute form of parietal pain is the rectus sheath
hematoma, found in patients with coagulopathies or
after strenuous exertion or coughing. The pain and
tenderness is severe and a mass is often palpable,
suggesting the possibility of an intra-abdominal
emergency. The diagnosis can be made with confidence
by ultrasound or CT scan which usually demonstrate
the hematoma within the rectus sheath.

3. Patients with intercostal or postherpetic neuritis may
respond to procaine injections over the painful
dermatome or in the paravertebral area of the nerve
origins. Transcutaneous nerve stimulation,
accomplished by use of a battery-powered, portable
pulse generator and electrodes which are applied,
empirically, over "trigger" points may also prove
useful.

PITFALLS

1. Chronic undiagnosed parietal pain often leads to
cancerophobia, frustration and depression. These
patients are studied repeatedly, often with invasive
procedures, which only reinforces the sense of
hopelessness. The 1st step in the diagnosis of

parietal pain is considering the possibility and performing the simple diagnostic maneuvers outlined above.

2. Patients with irritation of the xiphoid cartilage (xiphoiditis) may be misdiagnosed as having cardiac disease because of the high epigastric or low substernal location of the pain. The xiphoid cartilage often becomes more prominent in patients who have lost subcutaneous tissue due to weight loss. The cause for the pain is uncertain but may result from local trauma that is forgotten by the patient. The diagnosis is established by demonstrating the localized tenderness over the xiphoid and is usually sufficiently reassuring to preclude the need for therapy, although local infiltration with 1% procaine may be helpful.

3. Paravertebral procaine nerve blocks may be helpful in relieving intercostal neuritis, but the procedure should be performed by an experienced physician since pneumothorax can be a complication.

SUGGESTED READINGS

Harati Y, Niakan E: Diabetic thoracoabdominal neuropathy.
    Arch Int Med 146:1493, 1986.
Longstreth GF, Newcomer AD: Abdominal pain caused by
    diabetic radiculopathy. Ann Int Med 86:166, 1977.
Reuler JB, Girard DE, Nardone DA: The chronic pain
    syndrome: Misconceptions and management. Ann Int Med
    93:588, 1980.
Wright JT: Slipping-rib syndrome. Lancet 2:632, 1980.
Wyatt GM, Spitz HB: Ultrasound in the diagnosis of rectus
    sheath hematoma. JAMA 241:1499, 1979.

CASE 22: RIGHT LOWER QUADRANT PAIN IN AN ELDERLY PATIENT

A 68-year-old woman had been in reasonably good health except for osteoarthritis for which she took occasional aspirins or other nonsteroidal anti-inflammatory drugs. Her only surgical procedure was a hysterectomy at age 45 for uterine fibroids and menorrhagia. The day before admission to the emergency room she developed upper abdominal discomfort, nausea and subsequently vomited a small quantity of nonbloody fluid. Later that day she began to experience lower abdominal discomfort, more marked in the right lower quadrant. The pain had intensified, although no further vomiting occurred, and necessitated the hospital visit. Her temperature was 100.2 F, pulse 86, and blood pressure 130/75 mm Hg. Her chest and heart were unremarkable. Bowel sounds were present. Tenderness could be elicited in the right lower quadrant without evidence of muscle guarding or the presence of a mass. A digital rectal examination was unremarkable. The white blood count was 10,500 with 82 polyps, 14 lymphs, 3 monos and 1 eosin. The urinalysis showed 3-5 white blood cells per high-power field and 1-3 red blood cells per high-power field.

QUESTIONS (Please read the corresponding answer before proceeding to the next question.)

1. List 4 possible explanations for this pain pattern.

2. Which of the following diagnostic studies would you obtain?

    a. Obstruction series.

    b. Ultrasound.

    c. Upper GI and small bowel barium x-ray.

    d. Intravenous pyelogram.

    e. Barium enema.

3. If this were appendicitis would you expect vomiting to precede or follow the onset of abdominal pain?

4. What conclusions can be drawn from the patient's temperature when considering the possibility of appendicitis?

5. How would you proceed at this point?

ANSWERS

1. The following possibilities should be included in the differential diagnosis, although a number of others could be added:
    a. Appendicitis: Upper abdominal discomfort localizing in the right lower quadrant.
    b. Acute ileitis: Right lower quadrant pain and tenderness could represent an acute ileitis, even in an older patient.
    c. Right-sided ureteral stone: The urinalysis does not reflect this but the pain location raises that possibility.
    d. Diverticulitis: This process in a redundant sigmoid colon could lead to right lower quadrant pain and tenderness.

    Also consider Yersinia infection, confined perforation of a cecal carcinoma, intestinal obstruction and perforation of a peptic ulcer with leakage of gastric contents into the right lower quadrant.

2. a. Obstruction series: There was no abnormality noted.
    b. An ultrasound study was performed to evaluate for possible appendicitis. (The sensitivity of the procedure is said to be 75-85%.) There was no evidence of appendicitis found and no signs of renal stone disease.
    c. A barium upper GI x-ray was not performed in view of the lower abdominal localization.
    d. An intravenous pyelogram was not performed because of the absence of colicky pain or hematuria. However, approximately 20% of renal calculi are not detected by plain films of the abdomen.
    e. A gastrografin enema examination performed without air insufflation showed no evidence of diverticular disease. The appendix was not demonstrated. A contrast study should not be performed if perforation is suspected.

3. Vomiting usually occurs after the onset of abdominal pain. If vomiting is the initial symptom one should consider alternative possibilities.

4. The temperature is usually normal at the onset but gradually rises during the next 24 hours. It is unusual for high fever to occur in the absence of perforation. Fever which precedes pain should cast doubt on the diagnosis of appendicitis.

5. The patient demonstrates an inflammatory process in the right lower quadrant. It is not wise to "observe" the patient until more convincing signs and laboratory studies evolve, since these features may well reflect perforation. This patient was explored and an inflamed appendix removed.

PEARLS

1. It may be impossible to distinguish acute ileitis from appendicitis. If ileitis is found at exploration, the involved ileum should not be removed (at least 30% never proceed to develop the typical features of Crohn's disease), but an appendectomy should be performed if the cecum is uninvolved to prevent a recurrence of the same diagnostic difficulty.

2. The diagnosis of appendicitis remains a clinical one in spite of the potential value of diagnostic ultrasound or barium enema examination. A false-positive abdominal exploration rate of approximately 20% continues to be reported, but substantial reductions in unnecessary explorations may result in an increased incidence of perforation.

3. A retrocecal appendix often results in less localized discomfort and there is a lesser incidence of muscular rigidity in spite of advanced disease.

4. Although chronic appendicitis is not a reasonable explanation for a long history of recurrent lower abdominal pain, patients do occasionally experience spontaneous resolution of an acute appendicitis and develop recurring attacks which usually have the same features as classical acute appendicitis.

PITFALLS

1. Although muscular rigidity is a sign of peritonitis, a perforated pelvic appendix may not result in this finding. Indeed, the perforated pelvic appendix is an easily overlooked condition since the distended appendix no longer produces pain and the peritonitis may take 1 or more days to localize.

2. The incidence of negative explorations is higher in young women than men because of gynecologic conditions which may mimic appendicitis. A vaginal examination

can be helpful in distinguishing between these
possibilities.

3. Appendiceal perforation may result in obstruction of
    the fallopian tubes and thus contribute to infertility.

4. Although patients over the age of 60 account for only
    5% of all cases of appendicitis, the progression to
    gangrene and perforation is more rapid and the
    mortality is significantly higher than in younger
    patients.

SUGGESTED READINGS

Cope Z: Cope's Early Diagnosis of the Acute Abdomen, ed.
    17. New York, Oxford University Press, 1987, pp
    66-106.
Malt RA: The perforated appendix. N Engl J Med 315:1546,
    1986.
Puylaert JBCM, Rutgers PH, Lalisang RI, et al: A
    prospective study of ultrasonography in the diagnosis
    of appendicitis. N Engl J Med 317:666, 1987.
Samelson SL, Reyes HM: Management of perforated
    appendicitis in children--revisited. Arch Surg
    122:691, 1987.

CASE 23: LOWER ABDOMINAL PAIN AND RECTAL BLEEDING IN THE
OLDER PATIENT

A 72-year-old man has a history of hypertension, angina and
congestive heart failure which has been controlled by
digoxin and hydrochlorothiazide. He is admitted to the
emergency room with the complaint of left lower quadrant
pain of 4 hours duration and several loose stools
containing small amounts of red blood. Physical
examination shows his blood pressure at 140/100, pulse 104,
and temperature 100.5 F. His chest is clear. The
abdominal examination reveals reduced bowel sounds and
severe tenderness over the left lower quadrant. There is
no muscle guarding or rebound tenderness. A rectal
examination reveals blood on the examining finger. The
hemoglobin is 14.5 g% and the white blood count is 12,800
with 81 polys, 15 lymphs, 3 monos and 1 eosin.

ABDOMINAL FILM CLUE

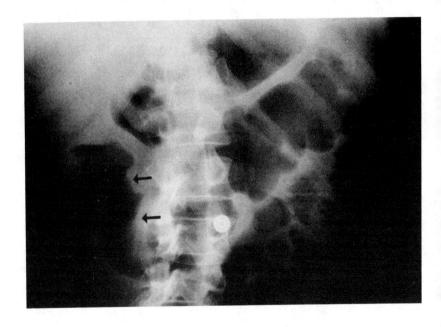

QUESTIONS (Please read the corresponding answer before proceeding to the next question.)

1. List 4 possibilities for this presentation.

2. What studies performed in the emergency room would be most helpful?

3. Should a barium enema or colonoscopy be performed?

4. What is the role of angiography in ischemic colitis?

5. Should corticosteroids be started?

6. How would you manage this patient and what complication would you be concerned about during the next several days?

ANSWERS

1. Diagnostic possibilities include the following:
    a. Acute ulcerative colitis can appear in the older
    age group, the so-called "second peak," and present
    with bloody diarrhea and abdominal discomfort. These
    symptoms are less typical for Crohn's disease.
    b. Diverticulitis is not usually associated with
    diarrhea and bleeding but the presence of signs and
    symptoms of an acute inflammatory process in the left
    lower abdomen should raise the possibility.
    c. Ischemic colitis should be considered in view of
    the abrupt onset of a colitic process in an elderly
    patient.
    d. An acute infectious colitis secondary to
    Salmonella, Shigella, or Campylobacter could result in
    bloody diarrhea and lower abdominal pain.

2. a. An obstruction series should be obtained to
    determine if a partial obstruction, air-fluid levels,
    signs of a pericolonic abscess or mucosal edema are
    present. This study showed evidence of mucosal edema
    ("thumbprinting") in the transverse colon. This is
    highly suggestive but not conclusive evidence for
    ischemia.
    b. A sigmoidoscopy without a cleansing enema should be
    performed. The enema may lead to mucus production and
    mild hyperemia which could be confusing if you are
    concerned about an acute mucosal process. The rigid
    sigmoidoscope was advanced to 15 cm and showed normal
    mucosa with red blood coming from above the
    rectosigmoid.

3. The normal rectal mucosa as assessed by sigmoidoscopy
    reasonably excludes an acute ulcerative colitis since
    the rectum is almost always involved. An acute
    bacterial infectious colitis usually involves the
    rectum but exceptions can occur. Because of the
    "thumbprinting" sign found on the obstruction series, a
    barium enema was not performed. However, if the study
    had been unremarkable a barium enema would have been
    appropriate, unless there were clinical signs to
    suggest perforated or infarcted bowel.

    Colonoscopy has also been performed in patients
    suspected of having ischemic colitis, particularly if
    the rectum is normal and the obstruction series is not
    diagnostic. This study should also be avoided if there
    are signs of perforation or infarction.

4. Although angiography can be helpful for the diagnosis
    of midgut ischemia involving the small and large bowel
    (thrombosis or embolism of the superior mesenteric
    artery or vein), it is not as valuable for ischemic
    colitis since this is usually small vessel disease. It
    was not performed in this patient.

5. There is no evidence to favor the use of
    corticosteroids when ischemic bowel disease is
    considered. An infectious cause has not yet been ruled
    out with certainty. (Stool samples were subsequently
    sent for culture, sensitivity and microscopy for ova,
    parasites and white blood cells.)

6. Ischemic colitis generally exhibits a changing clinical
    pattern. There are three clinical outcomes in this
    setting:
    a. The patient may progressively improve over the
    period of several days to a week or 2 (faster than
    would be expected with ulcerative colitis).
    b. The patient may proceed to infarction of the colon,
    demonstrating the signs and symptoms of peritonitis.
    c. The colitic process may lead to stricture which is
    often, but not necessarily, asymptomatic.

    Management should, therefore, be expectant, with
    frequent monitoring of the white blood count, vital
    signs and abdominal findings. Intravenous fluids
    should be provided and broad spectrum antibiotic
    coverage given since there is experimental evidence
    showing that the systemic effects of bowel ischemia in
    animals are diminished with antibiotic therapy.
    Evidence of increasing colitis should raise the
    possibility of infarction and consideration of surgical
    exploration and partial colectomy.

PEARLS

1. It has generally been held that the area of the splenic
    flexure is most vulnerable for ischemic disease, but
    the process occurs in all parts of the colon.
    Approximately 75% of cases involve the left colon, the
    transverse colon in 15%, right colon in 5% and, rarely,
    the rectum (in spite of its rich blood supply).

2. The distension which is associated with ischemia leads
    to compression of the mucosal vasculature and thus
    increases the ischemic process.

3. The finding of a colonic stricture in an older patient
    cannot be taken to represent the sequellae of a healing
    or previous ischemic episode without ruling out the
    possibility of carcinoma. There are several reports
    indicating that colonic carcinoma may occur in up to
    10% of patients who have had ischemic colitis.

PITFALLS

1. Digitalis and diuretic therapy appear to contribute to
    ischemic bowel disease by increasing peripheral
    resistance and decreasing the blood volume. Such
    therapy should be reduced or discontinued in older
    patients experiencing recurrent abdominal pain of
    undetermined etiology, since these symptoms could be
    the early symptoms of ischemia.

2. If surgery is required for patients with ischemic
    colitis who show signs of increasing bowel distension
    or peritonitis, efforts should be made to determine if
    there is a viable blood supply at the area of the
    proposed anastomosis. If there is uncertainty, it is
    prudent to perform a temporary diverting ileostomy or
    colostomy.

3. Ischemic colitis has been reported immediately
    following surgical repair of a ruptured abdominal
    aortic aneurysm. The colon appears vulnerable to
    ischemic necrosis in such patients due to hypoperfusion
    resulting from pre-existent mesenteric artery occlusive
    disease as well as the hemodynamic crisis associated
    with the aortic rupture. The colitis has also occurred
    following repair of a nonruptured aneurysm. A high
    mortality rate is associated with these cases.

SUGGESTED READINGS

Marston A: Intestinal Ischemia. London, Edward Arnold
    Ltd., 1977, pp 143-176.
Rogers AI, Cohen JL: Ischemic bowel disease. In Berk JE
    (ed): Bockus Gastroenterology. Philadelphia, WB
    Saunders, 1985, pp 1922-1926.
Schroeder temperature, Christoffersen JK, Andersen J, et
    al: Ischemic colitis complicating reconstruction of
    the abdominal aorta. Surg Gynecol Obstet 160:299,
    1985.
Scowcroft CW, Sanowski RA, Kozarek RA: Colonoscopy in
    ischemic colitis. Gastrointest Endoscopy 27:156, 1981.

CASE 24: ALCOHOLISM AND RECURRENT ABDOMINAL PAIN

A 52-year-old clerk has a long of history of alcoholism.
Six years ago he began to experience recurrent episodes of
upper abdominal pain which were diagnosed as pancreatitis
and which necessitated several hospitalizations. His
alcoholism continued and he now presents to your clinic
with the complaint of foul smelling diarrhea, weight loss
and increasing epigastric pain during the past 4 months.
An "oil-slick" was noted on the toilet water. Physical
examination shows a somewhat cachectic male. His liver and
spleen are not enlarged, there is epigastric tenderness and
the digital rectal shows light-colored stool which is
negative for occult blood. The hemoglobin is 11.5 g%,
white blood count 10,500, the amylase is 255 units (normal
to 100 units), the alkaline phosphatase is 160 units
(normal to 85 units), and the bilirubin and serum glutamic
oxaloacetic transaminase (SGOT) are normal.

LIVER ULTRASOUND CLUE

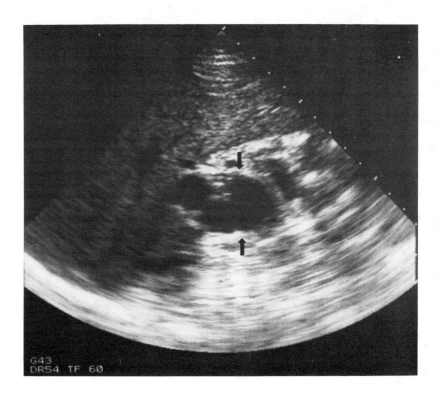

QUESTIONS (Please read the corresponding answer before proceeding to the next question.)

1. What feature of the stool appearance would suggest that the diarrhea is secondary to chronic pancreatitis?

2. Pancreatic calcifications were seen on the obstruction series. How does this affect your appraisal of the pancreatic disorder?

3. The ultrasound study also showed a 5 cm pancreatic pseudocyst (see Clue) and a moderate left pleural effusion. Which of the following studies or treatments would you perform?

    a. Endoscopic retrograde cholangiopanacreatogram (ERCP).

    b. Percutaneous aspiration and drainage of the pseudocyst.

    c. Surgical drainage (internal or external).

    d. Defer specific therapy for the cyst until the patient becomes symptomatic.

    e. Needle thoracentesis for the left-sided pleural effusion.

4. How might you explain the elevated alkaline phosphatase?

5. A stool fat collection shows 18 g excreted per day. What dose of pancreatic enzymes would you use for treatment of the steatorrhea?

ANSWERS

1. The description of an "oil slick" would strongly
    suggest the presence of neutral or unsplit fat. This
    is usually a sign of pancreatic insufficiency, since
    duodenal lipase would ordinarily split neutral fat into
    fatty acids and beta-monoglycerides.

2. Approximately 25-50% of patients with chronic
    pancreatitis are found to have calcifications.
    Although alcohol is the most common cause, the
    calcifications have also been found in
    hyperparathyroidism, hereditary pancreatitis and cystic
    fibrosis. No explanation is found in 10-30% of
    patients. There is no direct relationship between
    calcifications and exocrine or endocrine insufficiency.

3. a. An ERCP in patients with pseudocysts risks
    introducing bacteria into the cyst, thus leading to
    abscess formation. The study was not done in this
    patient.
    b. Percutaneous aspiration was performed and the fluid
    showed an amylase content of 25,580 units, suggesting
    communication of the cyst with the ductal system. Many
    cysts will remain decompressed, while others recur and
    subsequently require surgical drainage and internal
    anastomosis. This patient had relief of pain by cyst
    aspiration and decompression.
    c. Surgical drainage and internal anastomosis to the
    stomach or jejunum should be performed when
    percutaneous aspiration cannot be performed for
    technical reasons or the cyst recurs after needle
    aspiration. Continued alcohol ingestion influences the
    likelihood of recurrent pseudocysts.
    d. An untreated pancreatic pseudocyst may lead to
    persistent pain, "selective" portal hypertension
    secondary to compression of the portal vein,
    obstructive jaundice or rupture. The cyst wall should
    be allowed to "mature" for 6-8 weeks following an
    attack of acute pancreatitis, but plans should be
    directed toward needle aspiration or surgical drainage
    to prevent the above complications.
    e. Needle thoracentesis should be performed to
    determine whether the amylase is extremely high, when
    compared to the serum amylase, thus suggesting a
    pancreatic fistula with ductal contents tracking
    upwards and through spaces in the diaphragm. If the
    pleural effusion amylase is similar to the serum
    amylase, as was true in this case, the pleural fluid is

probably a "sympathetic" effusion secondary to the subdiaphragmatic irritation of the pseudocyst.

4. The elevated alkaline phosphatase could represent compression of the distal common bile duct by an edematous or fibrotic pancreas. An isolated elevation of the alkaline phosphatase is an early finding, but severe compression can result in jaundice and complete biliary obstruction. An ERCP in this case showed no evidence of obstruction, and a liver biopsy subsequently revealed evidence of fatty infiltration, probably secondary to his alcoholism.

5. There is no "correct" dose of pancreatic enzyme replacement. Sufficient enzymes should be given with the meals, or between meals if necessary, to reduce the frequency and discomfort associated with the steatorrhea. If the patient does not respond well to 3 or 4 tablets with each meal (use a preparation with a high lipase content), suppressing gastric acid with oral bicarbonate or H2-receptor antagonist can reduce degradation of the enzymes. The gastric pH should be maintained above 4.0 in order to prevent lipase degradation.

PEARLS

1. Although frank diabetes is present in only 10-30% of patients with chronic pancreatitis, an abnormal glucose tolerance test is present in over 70% of patients at some time in the course of their disease. Insulin-dependent patients may be difficult to control but there is a lesser frequency of retinopathy, nephropathy and vascular disease as compared to patients with genetic diabetes of similar duration.

2. The presence of splenomegaly, epigastric bruit and gastric varices should suggest "selective" portal hypertension. This results from compression of the splenic vein by pancreatic carcinoma, pancreatitis or a pseudocyst. High pressure builds in the splenic vein and flows through the short gastric veins to the fundal plexus and down the coronary vein to the portal vein. The bruit results from pressure on the splenic artery. Splenectomy relieves the portal hypertension.

3. Thirty to 50% of pancreatic pseudocysts following acute pancreatitis will resolve spontaneously within several

weeks of their formation, but this is unlikely to occur with chronic cysts.

4. The mortality rate for acute exacerbations of chronic pancreatitis (2-5%) is less than observed for episodes of acute pancreatitis (10-15%). Patients with advanced chronic pancreatitis are far more likely to die from complications such as diabetes, pseudocyst and malnutrition than from acute exacerbations.

5. Chronic pancreatitis rarely results from biliary stone disease since the gallbladder or common duct complications usually lead to surgery.

PITFALLS

1. The pain management of chronic pancreatitis patients is often difficult. It is best to start with the non-narcotic analgesics but many patients eventually become addicted to narcotics, either medically or elicitly. If necessary, it is preferable to use oral narcotics for pain relief than force the patient to search for parenteral drugs. Chronic pain, however, may be a sign of pseudocyst formation. An attempt to percutaneously aspirate small cysts may be worthwhile.

2. Prolonged observation of a pancreatic pseudocyst, beyond the 6 weeks necessary for cyst wall maturation, may lead to complications, such as bile duct obstruction, recurrent pain, infection within the cyst (thus producing an abscess) or erosion of the cyst into the splenic artery leading to a pseudoaneurysm, a surgical emergency. Although most pancreatic abscesses occur following acute pancreatitis, 15-25% occur in patients with chronic pancreatitis.

3. Patients with subclinical pancreatic steatorrhea will often develop overt malabsorption if gastric surgery is performed for the treatment of peptic ulcer disease. It would be prudent to consider 24-hour stool fat determinations in patients with chronic pancreatitis being considered for ulcer surgery, since the finding may influence the decision for surgery or the operative procedure.

4. Subtotal or total pancreatectomy and duct drainage procedures have a relatively high rate of complications. The painful exacerbations of chronic pancreatitis often subside with time, suggesting that

surgery should be reserved for those patients whose discomfort is severe and cannot be relieved medically. If surgery is required, a preoperative endoscopic retrograde cholangiopanacreatogram (ERCP) is required to determine whether resection or duct drainage should be performed.

SUGGESTED READINGS

Bank S: Chronic pancreatitis: Clinical features and medical management. Am J Gastroenterol 81:153, 1986.
Ephgrave K, Hunt JL: Presentation of pancreatic pseudocysts: Implications for timing of surgical intervention. Am J Surg 151:749, 1986.
Kohler H, Schafmayer A, Ludtke FE, et al: Surgical treatment of pancreatic pseudocysts. Br J Surg 74:813, 1987.
Lankisch PG, Otto J, Erkelenz I, et al: Pancreatic calcifications: No indicator of severe exocrine pancreatic insufficiency. Gastroenterology 90:617, 1986.
McClave SA, McAllister EW, Karl RC, et al: Pancreatic abscess: 10 year experience at the University of South Florida. Am J Gastroenterol 81:180, 1986.
Sarles H: Etiopathogenesis and definition of chronic pancreatitis. Dig Dis Sci 31:91S, 1986.

CASE 25:   HEARTBURN LEADING TO DYSPHAGIA

A 62-year-old woman has experienced frequent heartburn for
many years but has noted difficulty swallowing solid food
for the past 2 months. She describes the food as
"sticking" in the low substernal area. The heartburn seems
to be less frequent recently. There has been no
significant weight loss and she denies chest or abdominal
pain. She takes occasional aspirin for osteoarthritis and
furosemide 40 mg daily for mild hypertension. Physical
examination shows no significant abnormality in the chest
or abdomen. The rectal examination reveals brown stool
which is negative for occult blood. Her referring
physician had obtained an upper GI barium x-ray (see Clue).

UPPER GI X-RAY CLUE

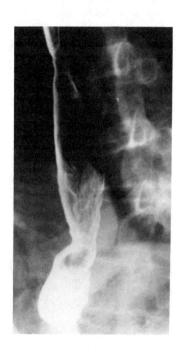

QUESTIONS (Please read the corresponding answer before proceeding to the next question.)

1. What is the reason for recommending upper GI endoscopy in this patient?

2. What are the criteria for the diagnosis of Barrett's epithelium?

3. What approach would you use for the esophageal stricture?

4. What dietary and pharmacologic measures would you outline?

5. Are pharmacologic measures more effective in relieving symptoms or improving the esophageal endoscopic findings?

6. How effective is antireflux surgery?

ANSWERS

1. Although a stricture is demonstrated on the barium x-ray, biopsies and cytology should be performed to rule out malignancy. The endoscopy can also determine whether Barrett's mucosa is present. The stricture in this patient was seen to occur in the midesophagus. There was a circumferential inflammatory reaction within and distal to the stricture.

2. Barrett's epithelium occurs in approximately 10-12% of patients with chronic gastroesophageal reflux and predisposes these patients to the risk of adenocarcinoma. The term "Barrett's esophagus" should be applied to the extension of the columnar epithelium into the esophagus for a distance of 2 or more cm above the esophagogastric junction. Although originally considered to be of congenital etiology, its association with chronic reflux is now well established. Three types of columnar epithelium have been described: gastric-fundic, gastric-cardiac and a specialized type with a villiform surface and goblet cells similar to that observed in gastric atrophy with intestinalization. The "misplaced" Barrett's epithelium is less resistant to trauma sustained by esophageal mucosa and is more likely to ulcerate or stricture (often at the squamocolumnar junction). Because of the malignant potential of this mucosa, the biopsies should be examined for evidence of high grade dysplasia, a potential clue to the presence or impending development of adenocarcinoma.

3. The esophageal stricture should be dilated in an effort to improve swallowing. This can be accomplished with the passage of mercury-weighted bougies of increasing size or the inflation of balloons of increasing diameter under endoscopic or fluoroscopic control. Both measures have a high degree of immediate success when combined with an appropriate medical program, but restenosis is common and the the procedure may have to be repeated at intervals, depending upon how soon symptoms recur.

4. a. Dietary measures should include avoidance of foods which can decrease the lower esophageal sphincter (LES), such as coffee, alcohol, oils, chocolate and mints, eating smaller meals, not lying down for 2 hours after meals, and elevating the head of the bed by 4-6 inches to reduce nocturnal reflux.

   b. Although the above measures may be sufficient for
   patients with heartburn without complications, patients
   with esophagitis should receive H2-receptor antagonist
   therapy given twice daily rather than a nightly single
   dose as used for peptic ulcer disease. If the response
   is not adequate, drugs which increase LES tone, such as
   metoclopramide or bethanechol, should be added.

5. Relief of reflux symptoms is often dramatic with the
    above program but the correlation with endoscopic
    improvement depends upon the severity of the
    esophagitis. Patients with isolated erosions have a
    6-week healing rate of approximately 78%, while those
    with more severe and confluent inflammatory change have
    a healing rate of approximately 25%. Smoking has an
    adverse effect on healing. The variability of the
    response indicates a need for continuous therapy in
    some patients in order to avoid the serious
    complications which may occur.

6. Before considering surgery for refractory esophageal
    reflux disease, consider whether your medical program
    is adequate. Perhaps a stronger dose of H2-receptor
    antagonist is necessary or the patient has not been
    compliant in terms of medication dosage. Several
    effective antireflux procedures are available,
    including the Nissen, Hill and Belsey operations.
    Their success depends upon the skill and experience of
    the surgeon and usually lead to an increased LES
    pressure and diminished reflux. Early postoperative
    complications include dysphagia (which may require
    dilatations) and the gas-bloat syndrome, resulting from
    the inability to belch after meals. Fortunately, the
    latter problem usually subsides with time. The
    Angelchik prosthesis, a silicone collar which is
    slipped around the esophagus just proximal to the
    esophagogastric junction and below the diaphragm, has
    also diminished reflux but the frequency of
    complications due to erosion of the prosthesis into the
    GI tract or its migration has led to diminished
    enthusiasm for its use.

PEARLS

1. The region of the sternum where dysphagia is located by
    the patient may indicate the location of the esophageal
    stenosis. For instance, food "sticking" in the low
    substernal area is usually due to an obstructing
    process in the lower esophagus, but food described as

"sticking" in the upper chest may on occasion be secondary to motor disturbances initiated by a lower esophageal obstruction.

2. The character of the dysphagia may provide information about the cause of the obstruction. For example, patients who initially experience dysphagia for solid food, then soft food, and then liquids show evidence of a decreasing esophageal diameter, usually due to carcinoma or gastroesophageal reflux disease (GERD). If the initial dysphagia is for liquids, consider a motility disturbance. If the dysphagia is episodic for solids with normal swallowing between symptoms, consider a lower esophageal ring.

3. Raynaud's phenomenon in association with reflux symptoms should suggest scleroderma. The esophageal symptoms, secondary to severe relaxation of the LES, may precede the dermatologic manifestations. Such patients should be placed on maintenance H2-receptor antagonist therapy since the symptoms are not likely to improve with purely dietary management.

4. Inquire whether patients who describe a "lump" in the throat experience dysphagia or cough while eating. High cervical lesions usually lead to pulmonary symptoms. Patients who can swallow normally but have a sense of tightness in the throat usually have no observable obstruction and are considered as having a globus reaction, spasm of the superior esophageal sphincter (cricopharyngeus muscle). This is a motility disorder but requires an upper GI x-ray with attention to the pharynx to rule out a neoplasm.

5. The availability of ambulatory 24-hour pH monitoring now permits correlation of chest pain with reflux, indicates the position when reflux occurs most often (erect or supine), relation of reflux to meals and whether the dosage of H2-receptor or sphincter tightening medications is adequate.

6. Most patients have solid food dysphagia when the lumen is narrowed to less than 12 mm in diameter. Benign tumors of the esophagus, such as leiomyomas, rarely cause dysphagia.

PITFALLS

1. GERD should be considered in children and adults with asthma, chronic bronchitis and unexplained chronic laryngitis. The reflux need not spill directly into the lungs since reflexes stimulated by regurgitation into the distal or mid esophagus may initiate bronchospastic reactions. This is often a nocturnal problem and can be best studied with 24-hour ambulatory pH monitoring. Failure to recognize this possible etiology for pulmonary and laryngeal symptoms precludes the possibility of significant improvement with medical antireflux therapy.

2. Metoclopramide is a useful drug for increasing LES pressure and enhancing gastric emptying. It is a dopamine antagonist and may result in fatigue and, rarely, dystonic reactions.

3. The most important nonpharmacologic antireflux measure is elevating the head of the bed, thus allowing gravity to reduce the frequency of gastric contents entering the esophagus. Many patients insist that they sleep on several pillows, but this is ineffective since patients usually manage to elevate the head rather than the chest and their position changes during sleep so that the elevation, if correctly applied in the evening, is not effective after several hours. Elevating the head of the bed by 4-6 inches or insertion of a wedge between the mattress and bed springs are the best approaches.

4. Infusion of enteral feedings through a small nasogastric tube or a percutaneous endoscopic gastrostomy (PEG) can be extremely useful for nutritional purposes. Aspiration via an incompetent LES has been a serious problem for some patients. The patient's chest should be elevated during feedings or consideration given to performing a percutaneous endoscopic jejunostomy (PEJ) to prevent reflux. A PEG can also be changed to a PEJ if necessary. If there is doubt as to whether pulmonary symptoms are due to refluxed enteral feedings, the sputum should be checked with a glucose dipstick. The high glucose content of the feedings will result in the characteristic color change.

5. Patients with carcinoma of the esophagus should undergo bronchoscopy to determine if there is tumor invasion of the bronchus. If this found to have occurred, the

patient has a significant risk of tracheoesophageal fistula if radiation therapy is given.

6. Potassium chloride tablets (and other medications with tissue-irritating potential) should be avoided in patients with esophageal strictures due to the likelihood of inducing further esophageal injury. Liquid preparations are preferable for such patients.

SUGGESTED READINGS

Harvey RF, Hadley N, Gill TR, et al: Effects of sleeping with the bed-head raised and of ranitidine in patients with severe peptic esophagitis. Lancet 1:1200, 1987.
Johnsson F, Joelsson B, Isberg PE: Ambulatory 24-hour intraesophageal pH-monitoring in the diagnosis of gastroesophageal reflux disease. Gut 28:1145, 1987.
Koelz HR, Rirchler R, Bretholz A, et al: Healing and relapse of reflux esophagitis during treatment with ranitidine. Gastroenterology 91:1198, 1986.
Lieberman DA: Medical therapy for chronic reflux esophagitis: Long-term follow-up. Arch Int Med 147:1717, 1987.
Reid BJ, Weinstein WM, Lewin KJ, et al: Endoscopic biopsy can detect high-grade dysplasia or early adenocarcinoma in Barrett's esophagus without grossly recognizable neoplastic lesions. Gastroenterology 94:81, 1988.
Wesdorp ICE, Bartelsman JFWM, Jager FCAH, et al: Results of conservative treatment of benign esophageal strictures: A follow-up study in 100 patients. Gastroenterology 82:487, 1982.
Winters C, Spurling TJ, Chobanian SJ, et al: Barrett's esophagus: A prevalent, occult complication of gastroesophageal reflux disease. Gastroenterology 92:118, 1987.

CASE 26: ASCITES AND A RISING BUN

A 58-year-old man with a history of biopsy-proven alcoholic
hepatitis 1 year ago is admitted to the emergency room with
the complaint of increasing abdominal distension. Physical
examination showed the signs of chronic liver disease,
including parotid enlargement, spider angiomas, palmar
erythema, hepatosplenomegaly, obvious ascites and bilateral
pitting edema of the lower extremities. Admission
laboratory data revealed Na 134 mEq, K 3.2 mEq, CO_2 30 mEq,
Cl 98 mEq, BUN 17 mg, creatinine 1.1 mg, bilirubin 1.9 mg,
alkaline phosphatase 68 units (normal to 85 units), AST
(SGOT) 68 units, ALT (SGPT) 51 units, total protein 6.3 g%
and albumin 2.9 g%.

A diagnostic paracentesis was performed shortly after
admission and showed a low protein and negative cytology.
The patient was placed on a 1 g/day sodium and
1,000 cc/day fluid restriction, and was started on
furosemide 40 mg twice daily and spironolactone 25 mg 4
times daily. His weight decreased by 14 pounds over the
1st 4 hospital days. On the 5th hospital day his BUN was
78 mg% and the creatinine was 2.6 mg%.

CLUE

On the 6th hospital day the patient's urine output was
800 cc, the BUN was 94 mg% and the creatinine was 3.1 mg%.
The urine sodium was 18 mEq/liter and examination of the
urinary sediment revealed no cellular debris or casts.

QUESTIONS (Please read the corresponding answer before proceeding to the next question.)

1. What are the possible etiologies for this patient's azotemia?

2. How would you define the hepatorenal syndrome (HRS) and what studies would be useful for establishing the diagnosis?

3. What are the clinical features of HRS?

4. List several proposed pathophysiologic mechanisms for HRS.

5. What therapy might be considered for patients with HRS?

ANSWERS

1. a. In view of the aggressive diuretic regimen coupled
        with salt and fluid restriction, prerenal azotemia
        secondary to volume depletion should be considered.
    b. Obstruction of the urinary tract by stones, tumor
        or (more likely) prostatic hypertrophy.
    c. Acute tubular necrosis.
    d. Any patient with severe liver disease who develops
        acute renal failure must be investigated for the
        possibility of the HRS.

2. HRS can be defined as unexplained renal failure in a
    patient with severe liver disease. Studies to
    establish the diagnosis should include an ultrasound of
    the kidneys and ureters to rule out an obstructive
    uropathy and examination of the urine for electrolytes
    and sediment. The urine sodium is usually low (<10
    mEq/liter) in both prerenal azotemia and HRS, due to
    avid sodium retention. In acute tubular necrosis (ATN)
    the urine sodium is usually high (>30 mEq/liter). The
    urinary sediment is clear in both prerenal azotemia and
    HRS and contains cellular debris and muddy casts in ATN
    patients. The BUN/creatinine ratio in HRS and prerenal
    azotemia is >30:1 and is usually <20:1 in ATN. The
    difficult distinction, therefore, is between HRS and
    prerenal azotemia, a differentiation which may only be
    made after an adequate trial of volume replacement,
    which should correct prerenal azotemia.

    This patient had been receiving diuretics which may
    have made the urine sodium determination less helpful.
    The diuretics were stopped and 2 days later the BUN was
    110 mg% and the creatinine was 5.0 mg%. The urinary
    sodium was then 2 mEq/liter after an adequate fluid
    challenge and the urinary sediment revealed no casts or
    cellular elements, all consistent with the diagnosis of
    HRS.

3. The HRS occurs most often in patients with alcoholic
    cirrhosis but has also been observed in acute
    hepatitis, liver malignancy, Reye's syndrome and fatty
    liver of pregnancy. It usually follows an event which
    diminishes the plasma volume, such as gastrointestinal
    bleeding, or dehydration from diuretics, vomiting or
    diarrhea. Ascites, hypoalbuminemia, portal
    hypertension and varying degrees of jaundice are
    usually present. Although these patients become
    azotemic, the mean creatinine is often <5 mg% and death

is usually a result of hepatic complications, such as gastrointestinal bleeding or sepsis. The mortality rate for HRS is over 95%, although there is a tendency to discount the diagnosis of HRS if the patient survives.

4. The proposed pathogenetic mechanisms for HRS are uncertain but all seem to be related to active renal vasoconstriction of cortical blood flow, medullary shunting and the presence of arteriovenous and portosystemic shunts. This is presumed to result from a decreased "effective" plasma volume (EPV). Total plasma volume is usually normal, although considerable sequestration may occur in the splanchnic circulation and in ascitic fluid. These events appear to decrease the glomerular filtration rate and trigger the renal tubules to increase sodium and water reabsorption.

The renin-angiotensin axis is stimulated by the decreased EPV and the hyponatremia commonly seen in liver disease, thus sustaining the renal vasoconstriction. The decreased EPV also activates the sympathetic nervous system, further potentiating renal vasoconstriction.

Renal prostaglandin synthesis has been shown to be decreased, especially vasodilating PGE2. Bradykinins and kallikreins, potent renal vasodilators, are diminished in HRS. Endotoxins have been shown to circulate in approximately 75% of patients with HRS and may potentiate renal vasoconstriction. Another possibility focuses on the liver's inability to inactivate a humoral factor(s) produced in the liver or present in the blood.

5. Treatment is primarily supportive since no single therapy has been shown to have a major impact on the high mortality from this disorder (approximately 90%). Correctable factors, such as dehydration and urinary tract obstruction, obviously require attention, but these patients probably do not have HRS. Efforts to increase the plasma volume include administration of albumin, reinfusion of ascites (either peripherally or utilizing a peritoneovenous shunt) and administration of renal vasodilators such as dopamine and prostaglandins A and E. The results of these therapies have been variable but largely unsuccessful.

PEARLS

1. The HRS is rarely present when the patient is admitted
    to hospital. The syndrome commonly follows some
    iatrogenic or therapeutic event such as diuresis for
    ascites secondary to severe liver disease.

2. The renal failure in HRS is a functional disorder
    related to liver disease and does not represent an
    anatomic disorder of the kidneys. In fact, the kidneys
    from a patient dying from HRS can be successfully
    transplanted into another patient with nonhepatic renal
    failure and will function normally. Successful liver
    transplantation in a patient with HRS will also reverse
    the renal failure.

3. The maximal resorptive capacity of the peritoneal
    membrane is approximately 900 cc/day. Therefore, in
    the absence of peripheral edema, diuresis of an ascitic
    patient without peripheral edema resulting in a weight
    loss exceeding 2 pounds/day occurs at the expense of an
    already compromised plasma volume.

4. Relieving tense ascites by paracentesis, with
    intravenous albumin replacement (10 g/liter removed)
    may help to reduce the pressure on the inferior vena
    cava and increase the return of blood to the heart.

5. The peritoneovenous shunt has resulted in transient
    improvement of HRS but patients usually succumbed to
    their liver disease. The rare patient with HRS and
    relatively good liver function might prove to be the
    best candidate for the shunt procedure.

PITFALLS

1. Nonsteroidal anti-inflammatory drugs should be avoided
    in sodium-retaining patients with cirrhosis because of
    the potential adverse effects of diminished renal
    protective prostaglandins. Lactulose should not be
    given to the point of severe diarrhea since the
    dehydration might trigger HRS. The role of
    aminoglycosides in the causation of HRS is unclear but
    their potential nephrotoxicity suggests the need for
    their avoidance, if possible, in patients with severe
    liver disease.

2. Since the muscle mass of patients with severe liver
    disease is often diminished, the creatinine clearance

may be lower then would be expected from the serum creatinine level. The glomerular filtration rate (GFR), therefore, may be diminished in the presence of a normal serum creatinine.

3. Sepsis should always be avoided in any patient but may be particularly harmful in patients with severe liver disease or early HRS since the effects of sepsis may exaggerate the vasoconstrictive features of HRS.

4. There is reasonable agreement about the lack of success for hemodialysis in HRS but the approach might be considered if the liver disease is potentially reversible (acute viral/toxic hepatitis or fatty liver of pregnancy).

SUGGESTED READINGS

Cade R, Wagemaker H, Vogel S, et al: Hepatorenal syndrome: Studies of the effect of vascular volume and intraperitoneal pressure on renal and hepatic function. Am J Med 82:427, 1987.
Davidson EW, Dunn MJ: Pathogenesis of the hepatorenal syndrome. Ann Rev Med 38:361, 1987.
Epstein M: Hepatorenal syndrome. In Berk J, et al (eds): Bockus Gastroenterology, ed. 4. Philadelphia, WB Saunders, 1985, pp 3138-3149.
Linas SL, Schaefer JW, Moore EE, et al: Peritoneovenous shunt in the management of the HRS. Kidney Int 30:736, 1986.
Zipser RD: Role of renal prostaglandins and the effects of nonsteroidal anti-inflammatory drugs in patients with liver disease. Am J Med 81:95, 1986.

CASE 27: A POSITIVE STOOL FOR OCCULT BLOOD IN AN ASYMPTOMATIC PATIENT

A 58-year-old hospital administrator presents to your
office for a yearly check-up. He has no complaints and has
been feeling well. His past medical history is significant
for mild hypertension for which he has been taking
hydrochlorothiazide. He does not smoke or take alcohol to
excess. Both of his parents died in their 70's with
coronary artery disease. Physical examination of the chest
and heart is unremarkable. His abdomen is soft with no
masses, tenderness or organomegaly. Bowel sounds are
normal. Rectal examination reveals no masses. The brown
stool is positive for occult blood.

CLUE

The medical student working in your office wants to know if
you wish to refer the patient to a dermatologist to
evaluate a 5 mm skin tag in the left axilla.

QUESTIONS (Please read the corresponding answer before proceeding to the next question.)

1. a. What foods are capable of producing a false-positive occult blood test?

    b. Is this test equally sensitive for the detection of the same degree of bleeding from the colon as compared to the upper gastrointestinal tract?

2. Would you study this patient with a flexible sigmoidoscopy and barium enema or with a colonoscopy?

3. What are the different types of colonic polyps?

4. What features of colonic polyps influence the likelihood that that they contain malignancy?

5. What are the congenital polyposis syndromes?

6. How should a polyp that is found to contain carcinoma be managed?

ANSWERS

1. a. Red meats and food that are high in peroxidase
content, such as turnips, broccoli, cauliflower and
horseradish, may produce a positive occult blood
reaction.
b. The guaiac test is based upon the peroxidase
activity of hemoglobin, thus explaining the greater
sensitivity (if the blood loss is equal) for colonic
bleeding since upper GI blood loss results in
degradation of the hemoglobin by acid and pancreatic
enzymes.

2. If the history reveals no upper gastrointestinal
symptoms and the patient is not taking nonsteroidal
anti-inflammatory drugs (NSAID's), a greater yield in a
middle-aged patient would be obtained by investigating
the colon first to rule out polyps and colon carcinoma.
Although the combination of a flexible sigmoidoscopy
and good double-contrast barium enema is a reasonable
approach, colonoscopy would still be required for
polypectomy if a polyp were found. Colonoscopy is more
expensive if the examination is negative, but is less
expensive if a neoplasm is detected since a biopsy or
polypectomy can be performed during the initial
examination. This patient had a colonoscopy which
revealed a 1.8 cm pedunculated polyp in the midsigmoid
colon which was removed easily with the polypectomy
snare. Histologic examination showed this to be a
tubulovillous adenoma with a focus of adenocarcinoma in
situ at the polyp tip.

3. Polyps may be attached to the mucosa by a stalk
(pedunculated) or broad based in their attachment
(sessile). Neoplastic polyps include benign adenomas,
malignant polyps and polyps associated with hereditary
polyposis syndromes. Non-neoplastic polyps include
hyperplastic (sessile, <5 mm, normal histology),
inflammatory (regenerating mucosa after colonic
injury) and juvenile forms (excess of lamina propria
and dilated cystic glands, usually found in children
less than 7 or 8 years of age).

4. Malignant transformation is most closely related to the
size and type of adenomatous polyp. Only 1% of polyps
less than 1 cm in size contain malignancy. Polyps 1-2
cm in diameter have a 10% malignancy rate and polyps
greater than 2 cm exceed 40%. Villous adenomas have a
higher incidence of malignancy at any given size
(50-60% of these polyps over 2 cm are malignant). When

located in the rectum, villous adenomas may rarely cause considerable mucus loss and hypokalemia. A pedunculated polyp has a lesser incidence of invasive carcinoma than a sessile polyp of the same diameter. Because of their malignant potential, all adenomatous polyps over 5 mm should be removed.

5. a. Familial polyposis coli is the most common hereditary polyposis syndrome. This autosomal dominant disorder has an incidence of 1:10,000 births. The entire colon is studded with adenomatous polyps which begin to appear in the 2nd or 3rd decades. Adenocarcinoma is usually present by age 40, prompting the recommendation for prophylactic total colectomy in the 20's or early 30's.
b. Gardner's syndrome is associated with multiple colonic and small bowel polyps and mesenchymal tumors, such as lipomas, fibromas, epidermoid cysts and osteomas. The incidence of malignancy is equally high, thus the same recommendation for prophylactic colectomy.
c. Turcot syndrome is a familial polyposis syndrome associated with malignant CNS tumors such as medulloblastoma or glioblastoma.
d. The Peutz-Jeghers syndrome consists of hamartomatous polyps associated with pigmented lesions on the lips, buccal mucosa and skin. There is a 2-3% incidence of gastrointestinal malignancy at sites separate from the hamartomas and a higher incidence of nongastrointestinal malignancies.

6. A pedunculated polyp with carcinoma in situ at the tip requires no further therapy beyond endoscopic polypectomy. If the tumor extends into the submucosa but the cut end of the polyp is free of tumor, conservative management is usually sufficient. If the carcinoma extends to the endoscopic resection margin or if the polyp is sessile and cannot be completely removed, standard colon resection is recommended. Patients with previous colon polyps should undergo colonoscopy every 2 years for surveillance purposes.

PEARLS

1. The clue in this case indicated the presence of an axillary skin tag, or acrochordon, which is associated with an increased incidence of colon polyps.

2. Approximately 30% of patients with 1 colon polyp detected by flexible sigmoidoscopy are found to have additional polyps when examined by colonoscopy.

3. Pedunculated polyps are more frequently found in the left colon, probably due to the effect of peristalsis "dragging" the polyp forward.

4. Oral iron preparations are often said to result in a false-positive guaiac test for occult blood. This is an uncommon finding in clinical practice and a "positive" stool from a patient on iron therapy cannot be ignored.

5. It is uncommon for colonic polyps to cause major colonic hemorrhage because the bleeding results from the polyp outgrowing its blood supply, thus causing oozing from the tip.

PITFALLS

1. Subtotal colectomy with preservation of the rectum to restore bowel continuity and avoid an ileostomy has been suggested as an alternative for patients with familial polyposis coli. Frequent sigmoidoscopic examination of the remaining rectum would seem reasonable but carcinoma may still develop with this approach, suggesting that total colectomy with ileostomy or a sphincter-saving anal pouch procedure are the operations of choice.

2. It was previously believed that almost all diminutive polyps (<5 mm) were hyperplastic. The increased frequency of colonoscopy has shown that approximately 50% of these polyps are adenomatous, and these patients should be placed into a colonoscopic surveillance program.

3. A significant number of patients with colon polyps or carcinoma have a negative fecal occult blood test. This procedure is an inadequate screening technique for patients at high risk for colon cancer, such as those with a strong family history of colon polyps or cancer, and those with a previous colonic neoplasm. Colonoscopy (or barium enema) every 2 years should be performed for surveillance purposes in addition to the fecal occult blood studies.

4. Endoscopic biopsies of colonic polyps are inadequate for the purpose of excluding carcinoma because of the significant sampling error. The entire polyp should be removed.

5. Thirty-seven percent of colonic polyps are above the reach of the flexible sigmoidoscope, thus the need for full colonoscopy to evaluate patients at high risk or with positive fecal occult blood tests.

SUGGESTED READINGS

Cholbanian SJ, Van Ness MM, Winters C, et al: Skin tag as a marker for adenomatous polyps of the colon. Ann Int Med 103:892, 1985.

Cranley JP, Petras RE, Carey WD, et al: When is endoscopic polypectomy adequate therapy for colonic polyps containing invasive carcinoma? Gastroenterology 91:419, 1986.

Giardiello FM, Welsh SB, Hamilton SR, et al: Increased risk of cancer in the Peutz-Jeghers syndrome. N Engl J Med 316:1511, 1987.

Lieberman DA, Smith FW: Frequency of isolated proximal colonic polyps among patients referred for colonoscopy. Arch Int Med 148:473, 1988.

Stryker SJ, Wolff BG, Culp CE, et al: Natural history of untreated colonic polyps. Gastroenterology 93:1009, 1987.

Waye JD, Lewis BS, Frankel A, et al: Small colon polyps. Am J Gastroenterol 83:120, 1988.

CASE 28: AN INTRAVENOUS DRUG ABUSER WITH DIARRHEA

A 38-year-old intravenous drug user is admitted to hospital with the history of increasingly severe diarrhea for 6 weeks. He has recently been experiencing 8-10 watery bowel movements per day with weight loss and anorexia. There has been no gastrointestinal bleeding and crampy pain is relieved by defecation. Physical examination reveals a cachectic male in chronic distress. His liver measures 11 cm in the midclavicular line, the spleen is not enlarged, the abdomen is nontender and bowel sounds are hyperactive. The rectal examination is unremarkable and the stool is negative for occult blood. Significant laboratory findings include an albumin of 2.8 g%, alkaline phosphatase of 230 units (normal to 110 units), AST (SGOT) of 75 units and ALT (SGPT) of 90 units.

CLUE

The patient is found to be HIV positive.

QUESTIONS (Please read the corresponding answer before proceeding to the next question.)

1. This patient is found to be HIV positive. What is your differential diagnosis for the severe diarrhea?

2. What additional studies would you require to secure the diagnosis?

3. What diagnoses would you consider in order to explain the liver function abnormalities?

4. What additional studies would you obtain? Should the patient have a liver biopsy?

ANSWERS

1. The diarrhea is voluminous and strongly suggests a
    small bowel rather than colitic process. Although
    generally a mild disorder in immunocompetent patients,
    cryptosporidium is one of the most common organisms
    recovered in AIDS patients with watery diarrhea,
    malabsorption and weight loss. The cause for the
    diarrhea is uncertain since small bowel mucosa is not
    disturbed, causing some workers to postulate the
    elaboration of an endotoxin.

    Isospora belli has been identified in 10-15% of Haitian
    AIDS patients and also causes watery diarrhea,
    malabsorption and weight loss. Although poorly
    responsive to antibiotics, several patients have
    responded to trimethoprim-sulfametoxazole, but a high
    rate of recurrence has been noted.

    Mycobacterium avium-intracellulare (MAI) may involve
    both the small and large bowel and produces changes
    which resemble Whipple's disease. CT scan of the
    abdomen may demonstrate significant adenopathy in these
    patients, a potential clue.

    In the absence of recovering a specific organism, AIDS
    enteropathy has been suggested as a cause for diarrhea
    and malabsorption. In some series, as many as 40% of
    patients with these symptoms have no specific organism
    recovered, but more recent studies suggest that a much
    higher percentage of specific diagnoses can be
    established if cytomegalovirus (CMV) is carefully
    sought.

    Parasitic disorders and common intestinal pathogens
    (Salmonella, Campylobacter) should also be considered.
    There is some evidence to suggest the possibility that
    HIV infection itself may be capable of producing
    mucosal disease.

2. Esophagogastroduodenoscopy and colonoscopy should be
    performed to obtain random biopsies and aspirate
    duodenal fluid, as well as exclude Kaposi's sarcoma or
    other diseases. A-72 hour fat collection (18 g/day on
    a 100 g daily fat diet in this patient) should be
    obtained, considering 7 g/day as top normal. A
    D-xylose absorption study to evaluate the proximal
    small bowel and a Schilling test to study the distal
    small bowel should be considered. Stools should be
    carefully screened for parasites and cultures obtained

for bacteria, fungi, mycobacteria and viruses
(if possible).

The duodenal mucosal biopsy in this patient revealed
the presence of cryptosporidium in the microvilli that
border the luminal epithelium. The treatment of this
disorder has been disappointing.

3. Ninety percent of AIDS patients, in one series, had
some liver biochemical abnormality at the 1st
presentation of illness. Over 80% of intravenous drug
users with AIDS had serologic evidence of exposure to
hepatitis B, with 45% reporting prior hepatitis or
jaundice, and cirrhosis was identified in 23% of cases.
Most patients had modest AST and ALT elevations (as
observed in this patient) and chronic active hepatitis
is uncommon. The considerations in this patient should
include hepatitis B disease (he was found to be HBsAg
positive) and granulomatous liver disease, in view of
the elevated alkaline phosphatase, such as TB, MAI,
and CMV.

4. Although some biochemical evidence of liver dysfunction
is common in AIDS patients, they generally do not die
from the hepatic disorder. Perhaps this represents the
role that the normal immune system plays in the
development of hepatitis in non-AIDS patients, since
the hepatitis B virus is probably not cytotoxic by
itself. The hepatic inflammatory response, however, is
reduced in the immunocompromised patient. A biopsy
could be helpful, particularly when granulomatous
disease or lymphoma is suspected, and was performed in
this patient, showing several nonspecific granulomas.
Biopsy of the culture was negative and a diagnosis was
not established.

PEARLS

1. Colorectal biopsies have a high degree of sensitivity
for the diagnosis of CMV infection. Rectal culture for
virus isolation is significantly less sensitive. The
characteristic inclusion bodies should be sought in
each biopsy and the patchy distribution of the virus
indicates the need for multiple samples. A negative
biopsy, therefore, does not exclude the possibility.

2. Although bacterial pathogens such as Salmonella and
Shigella as well as common parasitic disorders such as
giardiasis and amebiasis are found in AIDS patients,

their incidence is no greater than in non-AIDS patients with similar backgrounds (drug abuse or homosexuality). AIDS patients with diarrhea usually have a lower number of OKT4 cells than those without diarrhea. This suggests that the more immunosuppressed AIDS patients are more susceptible to gastrointestinal pathogens.

3. Malnutrition, as evidenced by a diminished serum albumin and weight loss, is as common in AIDS patients without gastrointestinal disease as in those with small or large bowel disorders. This suggests that diminished food intake and increased caloric requirements due to fever or inflammatory disorders also contribute to the malnutrition of patients with gastrointestinal pathology.

4. Although rare, cholangititis has been reported in AIDS patients and is another consideration in the differential diagnosis of cholestatic liver dysfunction. Involvement of the intrahepatic bile ducts is indistinguishable from that seen in primary sclerosing cholangitis. These patients may also have acute symptomatic acalculous cholecystitis. The common bile duct showed dilatation with or without stenosis with markedly irregular duct margins. The liver histology is not diagnostic but microscopy of the bile ducts and gallbladder often show superficial ulceration, covered with purulent exudate and subepithelia edema.

PITFALLS

1. Although a liver biopsy may be helpful in the differential diagnosis of cholestatic liver dysfunction in AIDS patients, routine biopsy is usually unnecessary in patients with mild AST/ALT abnormalities since the results rarely lead to specific therapeutic intervention or improved survival.

2. Failure to identify Kaposi's sarcoma by liver biopsy does not exclude the diagnosis since it is one of the most common AIDS-specific lesions found at autopsy.

3. AIDS patients with oral candidiasis may not require upper gastrointestinal endoscopy since they almost invariably have esophageal involvement and therapy is not influenced by the location or severity of esophageal involvement.

4. Upper gastrointestinal endoscopy, even if it demonstrates visceral involvement, adds little to the treatment program of patients with cutaneous or nodal Kaposi's sarcoma.

5. Unfortunately, AIDS patients may be difficult to study with gastrointestinal invasive procedures because of associated hematologic abnormalities, severe pulmonary and neurologic disease and sepsis.

SUGGESTED READINGS

Gelb A, Miller S: AIDS and gastroenterology. Am J Gastroenterol 81:619, 1986.

Gillin JS, Shike M, Alcock N, et al: Malabsorption and mucosal abnormalities of the small intestine in the acquired immunodeficiency syndrome. Ann Int Med 102:619, 1985.

Lebovics E, Dworkin BM, Heier SK, et al: The hepatobiliary manifestations of human immunodeficiency virus infection. Am J Gastroenterol 83:1, 1988.

Roulot D, Valla D, Brun-Vezinet F, et al: Cholangitis in the acquired immunodeficiency syndrome: Report of two cases and review of the literature. Gut 28:1653, 1987.

Schneiderman DJ, Arenson DM, Cello JP, et al: Hepatic disease in patients with the acquired immune deficiency syndrome. Hepatology 7:925, 1987.

Smith PD, Lane HC, Gill VJ, et al: Intestinal infections in patients with the acquired immunodeficiency syndrome. Ann Int Med 108:328, 1988.

CASE 29: ASPRIN AND MELENA

A 53-year-old presents to the emergency room with a 2-day history of melanotic stools and epigastric pain. He denies any history of peptic ulcer disease or gastrointestinal bleeding. There has been no recent weight loss, anorexia or change in bowel habits. He has been taking 6-8 aspirin per day for the past 6 days for a tendonitis in his elbow. He smokes 10 cigarettes per day and denies alcohol use. Physical examination reveals normal vital signs, with no orthostatic changes. There was minimal tenderness in the epigastrium and bowel sounds were normal. Rectal examination revealed black stool which was positive for occult blood.

CLUE

Nasogastric aspiration reveals coffee ground contents which are positive for occult blood.

QUESTIONS

1. What are likely diagnostic possibilities?

2. What diagnostic studies should be considered?

3. What is the relationship between aspirin toxicity and gastric pH?

4. How common is GI bleeding in patients taking aspirin and nonsteroidal anti-inflammatory drugs (NSAID's)?

5. How should drug-induced erosive gastritis be treated?

ANSWERS

1. Aspirin-induced gastritis, peptic ulcer disease and
    esophagitis. Gastric carcinoma, small bowel tumors or
    vascular malformations of the right colon would be
    less likely possibilities.

2. The passage of a nasogastric tube would establish
    whether the bleeding site is proximal to the ligament
    of Treitz. Failure to find blood in the gastric
    aspirate does not, however, exclude the possibility of
    bleeding from the duodenum without gastric reflux.
    Nasogastric aspiration in this patient revealed "coffee
    ground" content without evidence of red blood.

    Upper gastrointestinal endoscopy subsequently revealed
    multiple erosions and areas of petechial hemorrhage in
    the body of the stomach. The mucosal damage induced by
    NSAID's is often more prominent in the body of the
    stomach than the antrum or duodenum. An upper
    gastrointestinal barium x-ray should be avoided since
    the accuracy of the study is reduced by the presence of
    blood and clots and the barium precludes endoscopy or
    arteriography for many hours (or days).

3. Aspirin has a local toxic effect on gastric mucosa.
    The major damage from aspirin occurs when the gastric
    pH is <3.5. Aspirin has a pK value of 3.5 and at lower
    pH's most of the drug is in the un-ionized
    lipid-soluble state which can freely enter gastric
    mucosal cells. This results in decreased mitochondrial
    oxidative phosphorylation and ATP production, thus
    leading to cell death. The underlying capillaries are
    then exposed, leading to direct vascular injury.
    Hydrogen ion back diffusion, diminution of the mucus
    layer, decreased bicarbonate production and decreased
    local prostaglandin synthesis also contribute to the
    gastritis, but mucosal ischemia from vascular injury
    appears to play the most prominent role.

4. Endoscopic evidence of submucosal hemorrhage and focal
    erosions are seen in a high percentage of patients
    within 24 hours of aspirin ingestion. The normal fecal
    blood loss, as measured by chromium-tagged red blood
    cell techniques, is less than 1 ml/day. Aspirin
    increases the occult blood loss to 2-6 ml/day in
    approximately 70% of patients and a small percentage
    will regularly excrete greater than 10 ml/day.

5. Re-epithelialization occurs within hours after a minor degree of mucosal injury. Gastric erosions often heal within 48-72 hours if the offending drugs are discontinued. Antacids, H2-receptor antagonists or sucralfate can be used for several weeks but prolonged therapy is not necessary.

PEARLS

1. NSAID's are one of the most common causes of upper gastrointestinal tract perforations in patients over the age of 60, most of whom are using the medications as treatment for arthritis. Elderly patients also appear to be more likely to bleed while on NSAID therapy.

2. Patients are most likely to develop bleeding early in the course of therapy with aspirin or NSAID's. Gastric mucosal adaptation occurs with prolonged therapy.

3. Concomitant use of antacids or H2-blockers with aspirin will diminish mucosal damage by raising the gastric pH to >3.5 so that most of the drug remains in the ionized, lipid-insoluble form which cannot permeate the cell wall. Nonacetylated salicylates, such as salsalate, may have less gastric toxicity than aspirin.

4. The administration of NSAID's with H2-receptor antagonists or sucralfate may reduce the likelihood of bleeding, but studies at the present time are not conclusive.

PITFALLS

1. Buffered aspirin contains insufficient antacid to neutralize gastric acid. Therefore, the incidence of mucosal damage with buffered aspirin is no lower than that with regular aspirin. Enteric-coated aspirin appears to decrease the gastroxicity. There may be some benefit in using therapeutic doses of a liquid antacid with regular aspirin, but compliance is usually poor.

2. Aspirin-associated gastritis is poorly correlated with symptoms and may be "silent." One study of asymptomatic patients taking aspirin found that 20% had unsuspected gastric ulcers and 40% had erosions on endoscopic examination. Intermittent stool evaluations for occult blood may be helpful.

3. Epigastric tenderness, once felt to be a reliable physical examination sign of peptic disease, is a nonspecific finding. It may also be present in pancreatitis, cholecystitis and in normal patients with no GI pathology. Indeed, epigastric tenderness in thin patients often represents aortic sensitivity.

4. Corticosteroids have often been implicated in drug-induced erosive gastritis but the correlation of steroids with this disorder is not as clear-cut as with aspirin and other NSAID's. Although patients with rheumatic disorders using prednisone appear to have an increased incidence of peptic disease, patients with inflammatory bowel disease do not seem to be as susceptible. Perhaps concomitant medications, such as NSAID's, influence the mucosal toxicity of corticosteroids.

SUGGESTED READINGS

Armstrong CP, Blower AL: Nonsteroidal anti-inflammatory drugs and life threatening complications of peptic ulceration. Gut 28:527, 1987.

Dooley CP, Larson AW, Stace NH, et al: Double contrast barium meal and upper gastrointestinal endoscopy. A comparative study. Ann Int Med 101:538, 1984.

Graham DY, Smith JL: Aspirin and the stomach. Ann Int Med 104:390, 1986.

Graham DY, Smith JL, Dobbs SM: Gastric adaptation occurs with aspirin administration in man. Dig Dis Sci 28:1, 1983.

Lanza FL, Royer GL, Nelson RS: Endoscopic evaluation of the effects of aspirin, buffered aspirin, and enteric coated aspirin on gastric and duodenal mucosa. N Engl J Med 303:136, 1980.

Larkai EN, Smith JL, Lidsky MD, et al: Gastroduodenal mucosa and dyspeptic symptoms in arthritic patients during chronic nonsteroidal anti-inflammatory drug use. Am J Gastroenterol 82:1153, 1987.

McGuigan JE: Peptic ulcer. In Braunwald E, et al (eds): Harrison's Principals of Internal Medicine, ed. 11. New York, McGraw-Hill, 1987, p 1253.

Roth SH, Bennett RE: Nonsteroidal anti-inflammatory drug gastropathy. Arch Int Med 147:2093, 1987.

CASE 30: ASYMPTOMATIC ALKALINE PHOSPHATASE ELEVATION

A 53-year-old white female was found to have an alkaline
phosphatase of 587 units (normal to 110 units) on a routine
SMA-12 as part of a complete physical examination. The
remainder of the SMA-12 was normal, as was all other blood
work performed (CBC, electrolytes and creatinine). She was
on no medications and had no previous significant past
medical history. She had been feeling well, and denied any
bone pain, abdominal pain, pruritis or history of hepatitis
or gallstones. Physical examination revealed no
significant abnormalities. Repeat determination of the
alkaline phosphatase was 626 international units. The
patient was 9 years postmenopausal.

LIVER BIOPSY CLUE

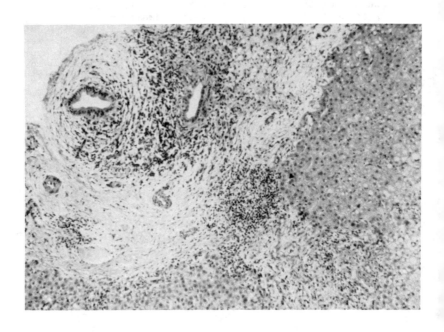

QUESTIONS

1. What are the sources of serum alkaline phosphatase?

2. What conditions can produce elevations of alkaline phosphatase?

3. What studies would be useful in determining the etiology of the alkaline phosphatase elevation in this patient?

4. What studies would be useful to determine the biliary tract abnormality causing the alkaline phosphatase elevation?

5. What are the common presenting signs and symptoms of primary biliary cirrhosis?

6. What are the histologic stages of primary biliary cirrhosis?

7. How would you treat this patient?

ANSWERS

1. Alkaline phosphatase is produced by the bone, liver, placenta and intestine. Certain tumors have been reported to synthesize an isoenzyme of alkaline phosphatase which has the same electrophoretic mobility as the placental isoenzyme.

2. Skeletal disorders such as osteomalacia, Paget's disease and metastasis to bone from other primary bone tumors, such as osteosarcoma, may cause elevation in the bone fraction of alkaline phosphatase. Pregnancy is a common cause of elevation in alkaline phosphatase due to placental production. In the absence of pregnancy and bone disease, most cases of alkaline phosphatase elevation are due to impaired biliary tract function. All types of liver disease may cause some degree of abnormality in alkaline phosphatase, including cirrhosis, hepatitis, drug-induced cholestasis, infiltrative diseases such as metastatic tumor, sarcoidosis, lymphoma or amyloidosis, as well as all causes of intrahepatic and extrahepatic biliary obstruction. The highest levels of alkaline phosphatase are generally seen with extrahepatic biliary obstruction (carcinomas of the pancreas, ampulla, common bile duct or duodenum, common bile duct strictures or stones and sclerosing cholangitis), primary biliary cirrhosis, and drug-induced cholestasis.

3. Elevations of 5' nucleotidase or gamma-glutamyl transpeptidase (GGT) are also elevated if an alkaline phosphatase increase is secondary to a liver disorder. In addition, the alkaline phosphatase can be fractionated to determine if the bone fraction is elevated. The GGT level was 6 times the upper limits of normal in this patient.

4. Dilation of the intrahepatic or extrahepatic biliary ducts by ultrasound or CT scan would suggest biliary obstruction. Cholangiography, either by means of a percutaneous transhepatic cholangiogram (PTC) or endoscopic retrograde cholangiopancreatogram (ERCP) would then be useful to delineate the cause. Viral serology is useful to diagnose acute and chronic viral hepatitis, which is usually accompanied by transaminase elevation. Liver biopsy might be required to diagnose infiltrative diseases of the liver. Antimitochondrial antibody (AMA) titers are positive (usually >1:80 titer) in 95% of patients with primary biliary

cirrhosis. Patients with primary biliary cirrhosis also may have elevations of IgM levels. There was no evidence of ductal obstruction in this patient by imaging techniques and the AMA titer was 1:320. A liver biopsy was performed.

5. Prior to the advent of automated blood chemistries, most patients presented late in the disease process with jaundice, portal hypertension, bleeding esophageal varices and other signs of liver failure. Since multiphase biochemical screening has become widely used, the diagnosis is now often made at a much earlier stage because patients are investigated when they may be found to have an isolated alkaline phosphatase and may remain asymptomatic for many years. The most common early symptoms are pruritis (47%) and fatigue (32%). Only a small percentage of patients now present with jaundice (13%) or variceal bleeding (9%).

6. There are 4 histologic stages in primary biliary cirrhosis. Stage 1 is called non-suppurative destructive cholangitis and is characterized by damage to the bile duct cells in the small portal tracts with inflammatory cells, lymphocytes and plasma cell infiltration. The hepatocytes are normal and there may or may not be granulomas present in the portal tract. Stage 2 is one of ductular proliferation in which there is a mixture of destruction of the damaged bile ducts from stage 1 and proliferation of new ducts. Stage 3 is characterized by scarring and fibrosis of the portal tracts. In this stage bile ducts become scarce and difficult to locate in the portal tracts. Stage 4 is that of cirrhosis and is similar to end stage liver disease of any etiology, with fibrosis, regenerative nodules and loss of the normal liver architecture. This patient showed stage 3 changes by liver biopsy.

7. No therapy has been proven to be effective for primary biliary cirrhosis. Cholestyramine is useful for relieving pruritus but does nothing for the disease itself. Steroids have not been shown to be useful. Although penicillamine effectively lowers hepatic copper deposition in primary biliary cirrhosis, it has not been shown to increase survival. Azathioprine, colchicine and chlorambucil have all been shown to be potentially useful in isolated studies, but require additional investigation. Liver transplantation should be considered for patients with liver failure or variceal bleeding.

PEARLS

1. Primary biliary cirrhosis is a disease almost
    exclusively affecting middle-aged women. Ninety to 95%
    of patients with primary biliary cirrhosis are female.
    The onset of disease is usually between the ages of
    30 and 65, with a mean age of 50.

2. Alkaline phosphatase elevation usually occurs early in
    primary biliary cirrhosis and plateaus shortly
    thereafter. The level of fluctuations of the alkaline
    phosphatase elevation rarely varies more than 20% from
    this level throughout the course of the disease.
    Changes in the alkaline phosphatase level during the
    course of the disease have no prognostic value.

3. Bilirubin elevation is an ominous prognostic sign and
    occurs late in the disease. Life expectancy after the
    onset of mild jaundice is 5 to 10 years, and only 2
    years after the development of deep jaundice.

4. Other autoimmune conditions are associated with primary
    biliary cirrhosis. Sjogren's syndrome is the most
    commonly associated condition as 75% of patients with
    primary biliary cirrhosis have xerostomia or
    keratoconjunctivitis sicca or both. Other autoimmune
    states associated with primary biliary cirrhosis are
    scleroderma, rheumatoid arthritis, CREST syndrome
    (calcinosis, Raynaud's phenomenon, esophageal
    dysmotility, scleroderma and telangiectasia), systemic
    lupus erythematosus (SLE) and autoimmune thyroiditis.
    Approximately 25% of patients with primary biliary
    cirrhosis have antithryoglobuin or antimicrosomal
    antibodies. Other antibodies found frequently are
    antinuclear and antismooth muscle antibodies.

5. Atherosclerosis is rare in patients with primary
    biliary cirrhosis, possibly related to abnormalities in
    lipoproteins, with high levels of high density
    lipoproteins (HDL's).

PITFALLS

1. Although positive, AMA titers are a hallmark of primary
    biliary cirrhosis but they are not specific for this
    disease. Modest increases of AMA titers can be found
    in chronic active hepatitis, connective tissue diseases
    and syphilis.

2. All 4 histologic states of primary biliary cirrhosis may coexist at the same time; therefore, a single small liver biopsy specimen may not be truly representative and may lead to inaccurate staging of the disease.

3. The antimitochondrial antibody is not cytotoxic to liver cells and therefore has no pathogenic role. The height of the titer elevation also has no prognostic importance.

4. The GGT has been used as a routine screening study for cholestasis, but the test may prove too sensitive and generate unnecessary biochemical and imaging studies if the alkaline phosphatase is normal. Its use should generally be restricted to determining whether an alkaline phosphatase elevation is due to liver disease.

SUGGESTED READINGS

Beswick DR, Klatskin G, Boyer JL: Asymptomatic primary biliary cirrhosis. A progress report on long term follow-up and natural history. Gastroenterology 89:267, 1985.

Christensen E, Crower E, Doniach D, et al: Clinical pattern and course of disease in primary biliary cirrhosis based on an analysis of 236 patients. Gastroenterology 78:236, 1980.

Dickson ER, Fleming TR, Wiesner RH, et al: Trial of penicillamine in advanced primary biliary cirrhosis. N Engl J Med 312:1011, 1985.

Kaplan MM: Primary biliary cirrhosis. N Engl J Med 316:521, 1987.

Lucey MR, Neuberger JM, Williams R: Primary biliary cirrhosis in men. Gut 27:1373, 1986.

Podolsky DK, Isselbacher KJ: Diagnostic procedures in liver disease. In Braunwald E, et al (eds): Harrison's Principles of Internal Medicine, ed. 11. New York, McGraw-Hill, 1987, p 1316.

Schaffner F: Primary biliary cirrhosis. In Berk J, et al (eds): Bockus Gastroenterology, ed 4. Philadelphia, WB Saunders, 1985, pp 3150-3176.

Van Thiel DH, Tarer R, Gavaler JS, et al: Liver transplantation in adults: An analysis of costs and benefits at the University of Pittsburgh. Gastroenterology 90:211, 1986.

CASE 31: DIARRHEA FOLLOWING BRONCHITIS

A 68-year-old male is admitted to hospital with a 4-day history of watery diarrhea, fever and lower abdominal pain. There is no history of similar illness in the past. There has been no recent travel outside the United States and the patient has had no recent contact with anyone experiencing a diarrheal illness. There is no history of inflammatory bowel disease. The only significant past medical history is mild chronic obstructive pulmonary disease (COPD) for which the patient takes daily theophylline. He recently completed a 7-day course of ampicillin for bronchitis.

Physical examination reveals mild lower abdominal tenderness without peritoneal signs. Bowel sounds are normally active. There are no intra-abdominal masses or organomegaly. Rectal examination reveals watery, brown, hemoccult-positive stool. Admission laboratory data reveals a white blood count of 12,400 with 81% polys, 7% bands, 11% lymphs and 1% monos. Electrolytes, BUN, creatinine, glucose, hemoglobin and hematocrit are all normal.

CLUE

Stool microscopy shows many white blood cells.

QUESTIONS

1. What is the differential diagnosis in this patient?

2. What diagnostic studies would be most helpful?

3. Is clostridium difficile part of the normal colonic flora?

4. What are the factors leading to pseudomembranous colitis?

5. What antibiotics have been implicated in the causation pseudomembranous colitis?

6. How is pseudomembranous colitis treated?

ANSWERS

1. a. The triad of abdominal pain, particularly in the
    left lower quadrant, an elevated white blood count and
    fever could suggest diverticulitis, although watery
    diarrhea is an uncommon presentation for this disorder.
    b. Viral, bacterial and parasitic infections should be
    considered in any patients with diarrhea disorders.
    The presence of leukocytosis and heme-positive stools,
    however, makes viral enteritis less likely, although
    cytomegalovirus (CMV) enterocolitis in AIDS patients
    can present in this fashion.
    c. Although inflammatory bowel disease is considered a
    disorder of younger patients, approximately 15% of
    patients experience the onset of their symptoms after
    age 50.
    d. Pseudomembranous colitis must be considered in view
    of the recent antibiotic therapy.
    e. Ischemic colitis must be entertained as a
    diagnostic possibility in an elderly patient with
    abdominal pain, white blood count elevation and
    heme-positive stools. Low flow or nonocclusive
    ischemic bowel disease is less likely in the absence of
    preceding dehydration or circulatory collapse.

2. Stool examination for culture, sensitivity, ova and
    parasites should be performed. The presence of fecal
    leukocytes would indicate a mucosal inflammatory
    disorder and would make toxigenic and viral disorders
    less likely. Stool examination for clostridium
    difficile toxin should also be obtained since
    antibiotics were recently used. An abdominal x-ray
    could show mucosal changes consistent with ischemic
    bowel disease ("thumbprinting"). A sigmoidoscopic
    examination would be useful to evaluate for changes of
    pseudomembranous colitis, ulcerative colitis and
    ischemic colitis. No enema preparation should be given
    since the irritant effect may lead to rectal mucosal
    hyperemia.

    The sigmoidoscopy in this patient showed mucosal
    hyperemia, friability and pseudomembranes and the C.
    difficile stool toxin was positive.

3. The organism is present in up to 3% of normal healthy
    adults, but the toxin should not be present in the
    normal state. In newborn infants, both the organisms
    and the toxin may be present in 30-70% with no ill
    effects, but soon disappear.

4. Since C. difficile is rarely part of the normal colonic flora in healthy adults, the initial event is considered to be a change in the gut flora, usually following antibiotic administration. C. difficile, which is ingested from the environment, subsequently proliferates, probably due to antibiotic suppression of organisms which normally inhibit C. difficile. Two toxins (A and B) are produced by the organisms and lead to the clinical syndrome.

5. Virtually every antibiotic has been reported to cause pseudomembranous colitis; however, ampicillin, clindamycin and cephalosporins are responsible for more than 80% of the cases.

6. The initial step in treatment is cessation of antibiotic therapy. This may be all that is required for resolution of the illness. More severe cases can be treated with oral vancomycin at doses of 125-250 mg every 6 hours, a program which is 95% effective. Oral metronidazole is also effective and much less expensive. Therapy should be continued for 10-14 days. Relapse rates are 15-20% with both drugs and such patients should be retreated. Other agents that have been shown to have varying degrees of success are anion exchange resins such as cholestyramine and cholestipol which bind the toxin, and other antibiotics, such as bacitracin, tetracycline and fusidic acid.

PEARLS

1. Antibiotic-induced diarrhea occurs in approximately 20% of patients on antibiotic therapy. C. difficile toxin is detected in 15-25% of these patients. The spectrum of C. difficile-induced colitis varies from mild hyperemia and friability to pseudomembranes, and may result in toxic megacolon.

2. Although the majority of patients experience their symptoms during antibiotic therapy, diarrhea may occur as late as 6 weeks after antibiotics are discontinued.

3. In addition to antibiotic treatment, C. difficile toxin elaboration has been reported after cancer chemotherapy and bone marrow transplantation.

4. Relapses of C. difficile disease are due to inadequate eradication of the organism with the initial course of therapy, and <u>not</u> due to selection out of resistant

species. Therefore, the original antibiotics, whether vancomycin or metronidazole, may be repeated.

5. Although proctosigmoidoscopy to detect pseudomembrane formation is usually diagnostic for this condition, a small percentage of patients will have normal sigmoidoscopic findings but the pseudomembranes may be found in more proximal segments of the colon.

PITFALLS

1. C. difficile toxin in the stool does not necessarily mean that the patient has pseudomembranous colitis. Only 20-25% of patients with positive toxin in the stool will have endoscopic evidence of pseudomembranous colitis.

2. Antidiarrheal agents such as diphenoxylate-atropine (Lomotil) should be avoided in this disease since "constipating" drugs may prolong the disease and possibly precipitate toxic megacolon.

3. Oral vancomycin is effective because it is nonabsorbed by the GI tract. The prohibitive cost of vancomycin suggests that uncomplicated cases be treated initially with metronidazole. Intravenous vancomycin has not been shown to be useful, although intravenous metronidazole has been reported to be effective. Oral therapy, if possible, is the preferred approach.

4. C. difficile should be considered a contagious organism and affected patients should be placed in enteric isolation. Patients who are immunosuppressed or receiving antibiotics should not be placed in the same room as a patient with a positive C. difficile endotoxin.

SUGGESTED READINGS

Bartlett JG: Treatment of clostridium difficile colitis (editorial). Gastroenterology 89:1192, 1985.
Chang TW: Antibiotic-associated injury to the gut. In Berk J, et al (eds): Bockus Gastroenterology, ed. 4. Philadelphia, WB Saunders, 1985, pp 2583-2592.
Gerding DN, Olson MM, Peterson LR, et al: Clostridium difficile-associated diarrhea and colitis in adults. Arch Intern Med 146:95, 1986.

Teasley DG, Olson MM, Gebhard RL: Prospective randomized trial of metronidazole versus vancomycin for clostridium-difficile-associated diarrhea and colitis. Lancet 2:1043, 1983.

Tedesco FJ: Antibiotic associated pseudomembranous colitis with negative proctosigmoidoscopy examination. Gastroenterology 77:295, 1979.

CASE 32: ODYNOPHAGIA AND PREDNISONE THERAPY

A 26-year-old homosexual male describes an 8-year history of systemic lupus erythematosus manifested by skin rash, arthritis and pleuritis, but his disease has been inactive for the past year on a daily dose of 10 mg of prednisone. Occasional heartburn is usually relieved with antacids. He has had retrosternal pain upon swallowing of solids or liquids of any temperature for the past 2 weeks. Antacids have not been helpful and he has lost approximately 5 pounds. He denies melena or hematemesis. The physical examination is unremarkable. The CBC, electrolytes, SMA-12 and creatinine are normal.

CLUE

Further study reveals a positive HIV antibody.

QUESTIONS

1. What are the diagnostic possibilities in this patient?

2. Are there any clues pointing to either major group of diagnoses?

3. What diagnostic studies would be of value?

4. What groups of patients are susceptible to candida esophagitis?

5. What treatment options are available for candida esophagitis?

ANSWERS

1. The major considerations must be peptic or infectious
    esophagitis. Patients with systemic lupus
    erythematosus (SLE) and other connective tissue
    diseases often suffer from gastroesophageal reflux due
    to abnormalities in lower esophageal sphincter pressure
    and esophageal peristalsis. Patients who are
    immunosuppressed, either by chronic steroid therapy or
    acquired immunodeficiency are susceptible to many
    infectious agents in the esophagus including candida,
    herpes, cytomegalovirus (CMV) and rarely
    cryptosporidium. This patient's presentation is highly
    atypical for a primary motor disorder of the esophagus.

2. Yes. It is most likely that the patient has a form of
    infectious esophagitis. He has had heartburn
    previously, probably related to his SLE, but is no
    longer obtaining any relief with antacids. Dysphagia,
    odynophagia, sitophobia (fear of eating because of
    pain) and weight loss, coupled with the lack of
    response to antacids or H2-blockers are common with
    infectious etiologies of esophagitis.

3. A barium esophagram in candida esophagitis would show a
    shaggy, irregular, finely nodular esophageal mucosa,
    usually involving the distal 2/3 of the esophagus.
    There may also be frank esophageal ulcerations.
    Although a barium swallow may be suggestive of
    infectious causes of esophagitis, endoscopy with
    cytologic brushings, biopsies and culture for
    specific organisms is the most definitive diagnostic
    modality. Demonstration of budding yeast and
    pseudohyphae on KOH smear is diagnostic of candida.
    Demonstration of intranuclear inclusion bodies is
    required to diagnose herpes or cytomegalovirus (CMV)
    esophagitis. This patient had a whitish, cheesy
    exudate coating the distal esophagus. The underlying
    mucosa was friable and ulcerated. KOH smears and
    culture were positive for Candida albicans.

4. Candida is part of the normal oral pharyngeal flora in
    35-50% and colonic flora in 65-90% of normals, and
    ordinarily is not pathogenic. Conditions which alter
    the accompanying flora or cause immunosuppression may
    allow candida to produce tissue damage. Patients on
    antibiotics, corticosteroids, immunosuppressive drugs,
    cancer chemotherapy or radiation therapy, as well as
    diabetics and AIDS patients, are at risk. The
    offending organism is usually Candida albicans,

although Candida purapsilosis, Candida tropicalis and Candida krusei have all been occasional causes of esophagitis.

5. Any offending antibiotics, steroids or chemotherapy should be discontinued if possible. Nystatin is usually the 1st oral agent used. Imidazole compounds such as ketoconazole, clotrimazole and miconazole are often used in patients who fail on nystatin. Systemic therapy with amphotericin B alone or combined with flucytosine is reserved for cases resistant to oral therapy or for patients with severe systemic candidiasis.

PEARLS

1. Oropharyngeal candidiasis is often an initial opportunistic infection indicating the presence of AIDS in high risk populations such as homosexual men, intravenous drug users and hemophiliacs.

2. Candida esophagitis is the 2nd most common infection in AIDS (31%) after pneumocystis pneumonia (58%).

3. The esophagus is infected by swallowed fungal organisms which then invade the mucosa, not by direct extension from oral thrush. This is exemplified by the absence of pharyngeal disease in many patient with candida esophagitis and the distribution of the latter in the distal 2/3 of the esophagus.

4. In severe cases, the addition of flucytocine may permit treatment with smaller doses of intravenous amphotericin B.

5. Complications of candida esophagitis include stricture formation due to fibrosis after invasion of the muscularis with candida, upper gastrointestinal bleeding, esophageal perforation and sinus tract formation which may lead to lung abscesses. Hepatic candidiasis has been increasingly recognized in recent years. Persistent fever in a neutropenic patient coupled with abdominal pain and an elevated alkaline phosphatase should suggest the diagnosis. Although ultrasound can be helpful in diagnosing the infiltrates, needle biopsy is required to establish the diagnosis.

PITFALLS

1. Although candida esophagitis has a typical x-ray appearance, barium esophagrams are normal in up to 25% of patients with the disorder. Upper GI endoscopy, therefore, is a preferred diagnostic modality.

2. Although candida and herpes have typical endoscopic appearances (grouped vesicles in herpes) the gross appearance alone is not accurate. Many patients have mixed infections which may have similar appearances (severe inflammation and ulceration). Cytology brushings and biopsies looking for intracellular inclusions are required.

3. Flucytosine should not be used as a single agent to treat candida esophagitis as there is a 12% incidence of resistant organisms to this drug.

4. Resolution of symptoms following treatment with antifungal drugs cannot be used as an accurate indicator of eradication of candida esophagitis in AIDS patients, since endoscopic evidence of infection may persist after many months of treatment.

SUGGESTED READINGS

Furion MM, Wordell CJ: Treatment of infectious complications of acquired immunodeficiency syndrome. Clin Pharmacol 4:539, 1985.
Kramer pulse, Burakoff R: Infections of the esophagus. In Berk J, et al (eds): Bockus Gastroenterology, ed. 4. Philadelphia, WB Saunders, 1985, pp 788-793.
Mathieson R, Dutta SK: Candida esophagitis. Dig Dis Sci 16:9, 1984.
McDonald GB, Sharma P, Hackman RC, et al: Esophageal infections in immunosuppressed patients after bone marrow transplantation. Gastroenterology 88:1111, 1985.
Tavitian A, Raufman JP, Rosenthal LE, et al: Ketoconazole-resistant candida esophagitis in patients with acquired immunodeficiency syndrome. Gastroenterology 90:443, 1986.
Thaler M, Pastakia B, Shawker TH, et al: Hepatic candidiasis in cancer patients: The evolving picture of the syndrome. Ann Int Med 108:88, 1988.

CASE 33: ULCERATIVE COLITIS AND PAINLESS JAUNDICE

A 39-year-old school teacher is admitted to the emergency
room with a past medical history of ulcerative colitis
since age 18. His colitis has been inactive and has
required no medications for the past 5 years. He complains
of fatigue and pruritus for several months, followed by
painless jaundice approximately 1 week prior to his visit.
He denies known gallbladder disease, hepatitis, intravenous
drug or alcohol abuse, or blood transfusions.
Physical examination reveals a mildly jaundiced man with a
liver measuring 14 cm in the right midclavicular line, but
no other abnormalities or stigmata of chronic liver
disease.

Initial laboratory investigation reveals: total bilirubin
3.7 mg/dL (normal 1.5), alkaline phosphatase 427 units
(normal 0-125), AST (SGOT) 38 units (normal 0-40), ALT
(SGPT) 51 units (normal 0-40), hepatitis A antibody
negative, hepatitis B surface antigen and antibody
negative, hepatitis B core antibody negative, ultrasound of
biliary system--no gallstones, no dilation of intrahepatic
or extrahepatic ducts, normal pancreas.

ENDOSCOPIC RETROGRADE CHOLANGIOPANCREATOGRAM (ERCP) CLUE

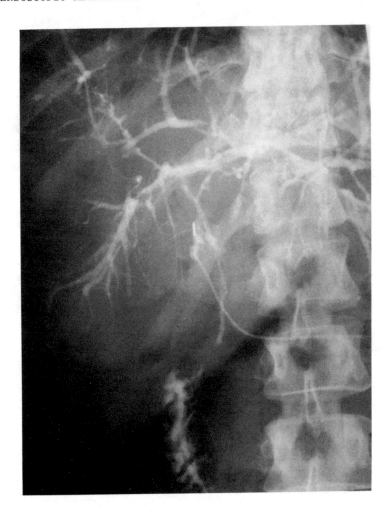

QUESTIONS

1. What biliary tract complications would you consider in this patient with a history of inflammatory bowel disease (IBD)?

2. What additional studies would be most useful in the evaluation of this patient?

3. What are the biochemical, radiographic and histologic features of primary sclerosing cholangitis?

4. What is the common clinical presentation in primary sclerosing cholangitis?

5. What other conditions are associated with primary sclerosing cholangitis?

6. What other conditions could be confused with primary sclerosing cholangitis?

ANSWERS

1. Cholesterol gallstones due to malabsorption of bile salts are more frequent in patients with ileitis than ulcerative colitis. Hepatotoxicity from sulfasalazine and fatty infiltration due to steroid therapy must be considered, but this patient has had no medications for at least 5 years. Primary sclerosing cholangitis must be considered in any patient with ulcerative colitis but is rare in patients with Crohn's disease. Cholangiocarcinoma has a higher incidence in patients with IBD than the general population. Other possible diagnoses include hepatitis, pericholangitis, liver abscesses and cirrhosis.

2. The liver function tests suggest a cholestatic pattern with very little hepatocellular inflammation. Hepatitis is unlikely in this patient and the viral serology rules out hepatitis A and B. The ultrasound results are not consistent with extrahepatic biliary obstruction from common duct stones or pancreatic tumor, thus the major considerations include sclerosing cholangitis or the various causes of intrahepatic cholestasis, which include alcohol, infiltrative liver diseases or primary biliary cirrhosis. An ERCP and liver biopsy are the most direct approach and, in this patient, showed histologic and radiographic evidence of primary sclerosing cholangitis (narrowing of the intrahepatic and extrahepatic bile ducts--see Clue).

3. Primary sclerosing cholangitis is a chronic fibrosing inflammatory disorder of unknown etiology involving any or all components of the biliary tree including the intrahepatic and extrahepatic bile ducts, cystic duct, gallbladder and pancreatic duct. The diagnosis rests on biochemical, radiologic and histologic criteria. Almost all patients have elevations of serum alkaline phosphatase of at least twice normal. Approximately 50% have hyperbilirubinemia at the time of diagnosis. Transaminases are usually normal or only slightly elevated. Cholangiography, either via the percutaneous transhepatic route or by ERCP, is essential to the diagnosis. There are diffusely distributed multifocal strictures in the intrahepatic and/or extrahepatic bile ducts and areas of dilatation between the strictures may produce a "beaded" appearance. The extrahepatic ducts are normal in approximately 20% of patients.

Histologically there are 4 stages of the disease by liver biopsy:
Stage 1. Inflammation of the bile ducts without spread beyond the portal space.
Stage 2. Tongues of connective tissue extend into the periportal parenchyma resulting in periportal fibrosis.
Stage 3. The inflammatory reaction extends between portal spaces (bridging necrosis) and is associated with septal fibrosis.
Stage 4. The last stage is one of cirrhosis which is difficult to distinguish from other causes.

The pathognomonic changes are found in the early stages with fibrous obliteration of the bile duct and their eventual replacement by cords of connective tissue.

4. Most patients (60-70%) are male and most are young. Two-thirds of patients with primary sclerosing cholangitis are less than 45 years old at the time of diagnosis. The majority of patients have had vague symptoms for more than 2 years prior to diagnosis. Fatigue, pruritis, jaundice and weight loss are the most common symptoms, but up to 50% may be asymptomatic at the time of diagnosis, their work-up initiated only because of abnormal liver function tests. One-half to three-quarters of patients have hepatomegaly, splenomegaly or jaundice at the time of diagnosis. The disease is slowly progressing with eventual evolution to cirrhosis and the complications of portal hypertension, hepatic encephalopathy and liver failure.

5. Fifty to 70% of patients with primary sclerosing cholangitis have ulcerative colitis although only 2-5% of patients with ulcerative colitis develop primary sclerosing cholangitis. Primary sclerosing cholangitis is also associated with other fibrosing conditions such as retroperitoneal fibrosis, Sjogren's syndrome, Riedel's struma and orbital pseudotumors. It has also been reported in association with pyoderma gangrenosum, chronic pancreatitis and vasculitis. Twenty-five percent of cases of primary sclerosing cholangitis are idiopathic.

6. The cholangiogram must be distinguished from other disorders which cause strictures of the bile ducts, such as previous biliary tract surgery, choledocholithiasis, congenital malformations and cholangiocarcinomas. Although the liver biopsy may share features with primary biliary cirrhosis (PBC), such patients are usually older women, have positive

antimitochondrial antibody (AMA) titers and rarely have
ulcerative colitis or abnormal common bile ducts on
endoscopic retrograde cholangiopanacreatogram (ERCP).

PEARLS

1. Although primary sclerosing cholangitis is frequently
    associated with ulcerative colitis, the 2 conditions
    have independent courses. Primary sclerosing
    cholangitis is not associated with exacerbations of
    ulcerative colitis and the disease may be diagnosed
    years before the onset of colitis or even years after
    total proctocolectomy for ulcerative colitis.

2. Ascending cholangitis is rare in primary sclerosing
    cholangitis in the absence of previous biliary tract
    diversion surgery. Infectious cholangitis, if it
    occurs, suggests the presence of a complication of the
    disease such as choledocholithiasis or
    cholangiocarcinoma.

3. The disease is of unknown etiology, although much
    information suggests that primary sclerosing
    cholangitis may be in part be due to altered
    immunologic mechanisms. There is a higher association
    with HLA-B8 haplotype than in the general population.
    In addition, there often are increases in circulating
    immune complexes and possibly anticolon antibodies
    which cross-react with bile duct epithelium. Decreased
    peripheral suppressor cells and increased B cells, with
    low OKT3 (helper)/OKT8 (suppressor) ratios in the liver
    and elevated OKT3/OKT8 ratios in peripheral blood have
    been described. Other theories involve viral
    infectious etiologies and biliary toxins derived from
    gut flora.

4. Although primary sclerosing cholangitis is a slowly
    progressive disease with average survival reported to
    be 5-7 years in earlier studies, a recent study
    suggests that more patients may be asymptomatic at the
    time of diagnosis and that average survival may be
    somewhat longer. Hepatomegaly and serum bilirubin
    greater than 1.5 mg/dL were poor prognostic indicators
    in this study.

5. Symptom benefit has been reported after combinations of
    endoscopic papillotomy, balloon dilatation of
    strictures and placement of biliary stents. Liver

transplantation is the most promising therapy for advanced disease with reports of 70% having 1 year survival. Primary sclerosing cholangitis is now the most common indication for liver transplantation at the Mayo Clinic and the 2nd or 3rd leading indication at other transplant centers.

PITFALLS

1. There are no specific serologic markers for primary sclerosing cholangitis. Antinuclear antibody (ANA), AMA, rheumatoid factor and antismooth muscle antibodies are almost uniformly negative.

2. No medical therapy, including cholestyramine, azathioprine, steroids, antibiotics and penicillamine, has been shown to provide more than symptomatic relief. Prolonged corticosteroid therapy will accelerate the osteoporosis found in patients with cholestatic liver disease.

3. Cholangiographically, it may be difficult to distinguish primary sclerosing cholangitis from carcinoma of the bile duct which may be multicentric. Complicating this further is the observation that 10-15% of patients with primary sclerosing cholangitis subsequently develop cholangiocarcinoma, making follow-up more difficult.

4. Patients with primary sclerosing cholangitis who have undergone total colectomy and ileostomy for ulcerative colitis have developed peristomal varices and bleeding. If colectomy is required in such patients, consideration should be given to an ileoanal anastomosis.

SUGGESTED READINGS

Chapman RW, Cottone M, Selby WS, et al: Serum autoantibodies, ulcerative colitis and primary sclerosing cholangitis. Gut 27:86, 1986.

Helzberg JH,Peterson JM, Boyer JL: Improved survival with primary sclerosing cholangitis: A review of clinicopathologic features and comparisons of symptomatic and asymptomatic patients. Gastroenterology 92:1869, 1987.

LaRusso NF, Weisner RH, Ludwig J, et al: Primary
    sclerosing cholangitis. N Engl J Med 310:899, 1984.
Lefkowitch JH, Martin EL: Primary sclerosing cholangitis.
    In Popper H, Schaffner F (eds): Progress in Liver
    Disease, ed. 8. New York, Grune & Stratton, 1986, pp
    557-380.
MacCarty RL, LaRusso NF, Weisner RH, et al: Primary
    sclerosing cholangitis. Findings on cholangiography
    and pancreatography. Radiology 149:39, 1983.
Mir-Madjlessi SH, Farmer RG, Sivak MV: Bile duct carcinoma
    in patients with ulcerative colitis. Relationship to
    sclerosing cholangitis: Report of six cases and review
    of the literature. Dig Dis Sci 32:145, 1987.
Schafner F: Sclerosing cholangitis. In Berk JE (ed):
    Bockus Gastroenterology, ed. 4. Philadelphia, WB
    Saunders, 1985, pp 788-793.
Wiesner RH, LaRusso NF, Dozoid RR, et al: Peristomal
    varices after proctocolectomy in patients with primary
    sclerosing cholangitis. Gastroenterology 90:316, 1986.

CASE 34: DIARRHEA FOLLOWING A CAMPING TRIP

A 38-year-old architect presents to your office with a
3-week history of crampy abdominal pain, flatulence,
diarrhea and a weight loss of approximately 6 pounds. She
has no history of previous gastrointestinal problems and
has otherwise been reasonably well. The stools are watery
and sometimes greasy, with a frequency of 8-10 movements
daily. There has been no blood in the stool. She and her
husband had been on a 7-day camping trip in the Pacific
Northwest 5 weeks ago during which time they both were
well. The patient is afebrile and other vital signs are
normal. The abdomen is soft, nontender and without masses.
Bowel sounds are normal. Rectal examination reveals
watery, light brown, heme-negative stool. A CBC and
routine biochemical studies were performed by another
physician and were unremarkable.

UPPER GI BARIUM CLUE

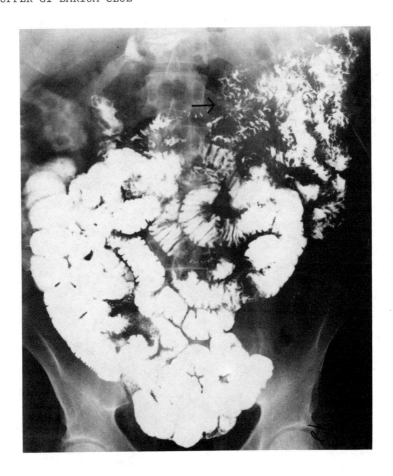

QUESTIONS

1. a. What would make ulcerative colitis an unlikely diagnosis?

   b. Is Crohn's disease consistent with this clinical picture?

   c. What bacteriologic disorders could produce this clinical picture?

   d. What parasitic diseases would you consider?

2. If you suspect giardiasis, what additional studies would you obtain?

3. a. Untreated, how long might this patient's symptoms continue?

   b. Is malabsorption a feature of giardiasis?

4. Who is susceptible to Giardia infection?

5. How would you treat this patient?

ANSWERS

1. a. Occult blood-negative watery diarrhea would be an
        unlikely finding in ulcerative colitis. A
        sigmoidoscopy without enema preparation should be
        performed when inflammatory bowel disease or infectious
        possibilities are considered. The examination showed
        normal mucosa.
    b. Crohn's disease could produce watery diarrhea but
        leukocytosis and some abdominal tenderness would be
        anticipated in the presence of these symptoms. An
        upper gastrointestinal and small bowel x-ray was
        performed (after the stools had been examined) and this
        revealed increased secretions in the duodenum and
        proximal jejunum.
    c. Cytopathogenic bacteria, such as Campylobacter,
        Salmonella and Shigella, would usually give rise to
        occult blood in the stool, but stool cultures should be
        obtained. (These studies showed no pathogenic
        bacteria.)
    d. Amebiasis and giardiasis are the most likely
        parasitic disorders to consider in this setting. The
        absence of leukocytosis and occult blood in the stool
        would suggest giardiasis, but the stool examination for
        ova and parasites was negative.

2. Stool examination for Giardia cysts or trophozoites may
    only be positive in approximately 50% of cases, even
    with 3 separate stool specimens. Stools should be
    examined as freshly as possible, since long delays
    decrease the diagnostic yield. Since the organism
    inhabits the intervillous spaces in the unstirred layer
    of the duodenal and jejunal mucosa, examination of the
    proximal small bowel fluid or small bowel biopsy should
    be the next step if the stool microscopy is negative.
    This can be accomplished by an Enterotest, consisting
    of a microscopic examination (for trophozoites) of a
    nylon string that has passed into the duodenum with the
    help of a gelatin capsule affixed to the end. Another
    alternative would be endoscopic aspiration of small
    bowel secretions and biopsy with examination of the
    specimens for Giardia trophozoites. Endoscopic
    aspiration of duodenal secretions in this case revealed
    many Giardia organisms.

3. a. The acute symptoms usually subside by 3-4 weeks.
        Of importance is the finding that some patients enter a
        chronic phase which may last a year or more. The
        symptoms are flatulence, intermittent diarrhea and
        crampy pain.

b. Malabsorption is a common finding during the acute symptoms. Vitamin B-12, D-xylose and fat malabsorption have been described. Patients with severe Giardia infestation may also have bacterial colonization of the proximal small bowel.

4. Giardiasis is more common in young children due to spread within day care centers. Campers in endemic wilderness areas who drink stream water, homosexual males and visitors to endemic urban areas such as Leningrad are at risk. Patients with numerous immunodeficiency conditions associated with IgA deficiency are also susceptible. Strain variation in the pathogenicity of Giardia infection has been demonstrated.

5. The 2 most commonly used drugs are quinacrine hydrochloride and metronidazole. Quinacrine, 100 mg p.o. t.i.d. for 7 days, is approximately 95% effective in eradicating the parasite but side effects such as nausea, headaches and dizziness are common. Metronidazole, 250 mg t.i.d. for 7 days, is 85-90% effective, with less side effects than quinacrine, but relapses may be more frequent. There is some concern regarding using metronidazole, a mutagenic drug in laboratory animals, for young children, but the risk of carcinogenicity in humans is not yet apparent.

PEARLS

1. Giardia is the most common cause of water bourne outbreaks of diarrhea in the United States.

2. In endemic areas breast feeding may be protective for infants, possibly due to specific anti-Giardia IgA antibodies in breast milk.

3. Although a travel history is usually sought in patients with giardiasis, as many as 1/2 of affected adult patients have no obvious risk factor. Therefore, the absence of a travel history from a patient with diarrhea should not dissuade you from the consideration of giardiasis.

4. There is promising experimental work with an enzyme-linked immunosorbent assay (ELISA) for detection of serum IgM and IgG antibodies against Giardia. This may help to increase the diagnostic frequency.

5. Boiling water for 5-10 minutes in endemic areas is
    sufficient to kill any cysts which may be present.

PITFALLS

1. Relapses of giardiasis may occur up to 2 months after
    treatment is discontinued, therefore patients should be
    followed closely after treatment.

2. Giardia cysts are resistant to the levels of chlorine
    normally used in water purification systems. This is a
    more significant problem in areas of poor sanitation.

3. No prophylactic antibiotic regimen has been shown to be
    effective for the prevention of Giardia infection
    during travel to endemic areas. The only effective
    prevention is to avoid contaminated food and to boil
    the water.

4. Giardiasis in pregnancy is a particularly difficult
    problem. Quinacrine is not recommended in pregnancy
    and metronidazole is contraindicated in the 1st
    trimester. If the disease is mild, conservative
    measures and rehydration are recommended for such
    patients.

SUGGESTED READINGS

Brandborg LL: Giardiasis and traveler's diarrhea.
    Gastroenterology 78:1602, 1980.
Cantey JR: Infectious diarrhea: Pathogenesis and risk
    factors. Am J Med 78(Suppl 6B):65, 1985.
Chester AC, Macmurray FG, Restifo MD, et al: Giardiasis as
    a chronic disease. Dig Dis Sci 30:215, 1985.
DuPont HL, Sullivan PS: Giardiasis: The clinical
    spectrum, diagnosis and therapy. Ped Infect Dis 5(1
    Suppl):S131, 1986.
Goka AKJ, Mathan VI, Rolston DDK, et al: Diagnosis of
    giardiasis by specific IgM antibody enzyme-linked
    immunosorbent assay. Lancet 2:184, 1986.
Monroe LS: Gastrointestinal parasites. In Berk J, et al
    (eds): Bockus Gastroenterology, ed. 4. Philadelphia,
    WB Saunders, 1985, pp 4278-4282.
Nash TE, Herrington DA, Losonsky GA, et al: Experimental
    human infections with Giardia lamblia. J Infect Dis
    156:974, 1987.

Plorde JL: Giardiasis.   In Braunwald E, et al (eds):
Harrison's Principles of Internal Medicine, ed. 11.
New York, McGraw Hill, 1987, pp 800-801.

CASE 35: EPIGASTRIC PAIN, FEVER AND JAUNDICE

A 73-year-old female presents to the emergency room with
the chief complaint of recurrent episodes of epigastric
pain during the past 9 months, but fever and jaundice have,
for the 1st time, occurred and persisted for 5 days. There
is no history of blood transfusions, hepatitis or
alcoholism. The patient takes no medication. Her past
medical history is essentially negative with the exception
of an uncomplicated cholecystectomy 8 years ago after an
episode of cholecystitis.

Physical examination reveals a mildly jaundiced elderly
woman who otherwise appears well. Abdominal examination
reveals no significant tenderness, masses or organomegaly.
There are no stigmata of chronic liver disease. Her
temperature is 100 F and other vital signs are stable.
Laboratory data reveals: white blood count 12,400 with 85%
polys, 10% bands and 5% lymphs; bilirubin 4.9 mg%, alkaline
phosphatase 368 units (normal to 115 units); AST (SGOT) 320
units, ALT (SGPT) 357 units, and the prothrombin time was
normal. An ultrasound of the biliary tract reveals a
dilated common bile duct with no visible stones.

PERCUTANEOUS TRANSHEPATIC CHOLANGIOGRAM (PTC) CLUE

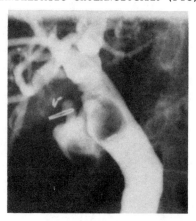

QUESTIONS

1. What features of the history and physical examination
    would assist in distinguishing between benign and
    malignant hepatobiliary disease?

2. A percutaneous transhepatic cholangiogram (PTC) showed
    evidence of a large ductal stone with partial
    obstruction and dilatation of the common bile duct (see
    Clue). How can you explain the presence of the stone?

3. How do you explain the elevated SGOT and SGPT?

4. If common duct calculi are suspected, what diagnostic
    and therapeutic measures should be considered?

5. List three complications of unoperated common duct
    calculi.

ANSWERS

1. The symptoms have recurred for 9 months but the patient
    appears well, with no evidence of weight loss or
    abdominal mass. This prolonged episodic course would
    be unusual for hepatic or pancreatic malignancy.

2. Approximately 10% of patients with gallbladder calculi
    are found to have common duct stones as well. The
    detection of postcholecystectomy choledocholithiasis
    raises the following possibilities:
    a. Stones were present in the common duct but not
    detected at the time of the cholecystectomy.
    b. Gallstones slipped into the common duct during
    manipulation of the gallbladder during surgery.
    c. The ductal stones formed subsequent to the surgery.
    This is more likely to occur in countries where ductal
    parasites, such as ascaris, are encountered. Any
    process which causes ductal stasis, such as stricture
    or compression of the duct by the pancreas, could lead
    to the formation of "primary" bile duct stones.

3. Although uncomplicated biliary obstruction usually
    results in normal or slightly elevated SGOT and SGPT,
    ascending cholangitis can give rise to considerable
    (over 300 units) transaminase elevations. Cholangitis
    is more likely to occur in the presence of common duct
    stone disease, in which the bile is infected in more
    than 1/2 the patients, than in malignant obstruction.
    Fluctuating fever, transaminase levels and bilirubin
    are highly suggestive of choledocholithiasis.

4. An ultrasound study is generally the best initial
    study, since duct dilatation can be evaluated and a
    bile duct calculus may be identified. Although
    patients with life-threatening infection have been
    treated with surgical biliary drainage procedures, the
    operative mortality can be considerable in acute
    suppurative cholangitis. ERCP should be considered if
    the endoscopist is prepared to utilize techniques, such
    as stone baskets and papillotomy, to facilitate the
    elimination of the stones. These ampullary procedures
    have a complication rate of 8-10% and include bleeding,
    sepsis, pancreatitis or duodenal perforation, with a
    mortality rate of approximately 1%, although still
    safer than surgery. PTC also permits entrance to the
    biliary tree, bile drainage and the use of stone
    baskets for fracturing the calculi. Antibiotic
    coverage is required during both procedures, ampicillin
    plus an aminoglycoside or a 2nd-generation penicillin

such as mezlocillin. If the calculi cannot be removed
with ERCP or PTC, infusion of the common duct with
monooctanoin or methyl tertiarybutyl ether may lead to
stone dissolution or sufficient softening to facilitate
removal. Lithotripsy techniques are being used for the
disintegration of gallstones and this approach may
prove helpful, after further experience, in the
management of choledocholithiasis.

5. a. Ascending cholangitis leading to multiple liver
abscesses (the most common cause for liver abscess in
the northeastern U.S.).
b. Stricture of the distal common bile duct due to
mechanical irritation from the calculi.
c. Pancreatitis secondary to the presence of the
common duct calculi and the high frequency of infected
bile in such patients. Patients with a history of
pancreatitis associated with biliary tract calculi have
been found to frequently pass small calculi in their
stool, suggesting that stone fragments may be passing
through the ampulla more frequently than clinically
suspected.

PEARLS

1. A patient with clinical evidence of obstructive
    jaundice and a history of cholecystectomy should be
    asked whether a tube drained bile into a bag for 7-10
    days following the surgery, indicating that a bile duct
    exploration had been performed, since previous common
    bile duct manipulation is a common cause of bile duct
    strictures.

2. Although jaundice is more common in choledocholithiasis
    (75%) than cholecystitis (25%), the pain patterns may
    be quite similar.

3. Escherichia coli is the most frequently found biliary
    organism in ascending cholangitis. Klebsiella,
    enterococcus, Pseudomonas and enterobacter cause most
    of the remaining cases. Infection of bile with
    anaerobes, such as Bacteroides fragilis and Clostridium
    perfringens is rare. Bile cultures may reveal multiple
    organisms in up to 80% of patients with ascending
    cholangitis and common duct stones.

4. Although a distended gallbladder associated with
    extrahepatic jaundice (Courvoisier gallbladder) is
    considered to be a sign of malignant biliary

   obstruction, approximately 15% of patients with
   choledocholithiasis are found to have clinical
   gallbladder distension and as many as 40% have the
   finding at surgery.

5. Cholangiocarcinoma is a long-term complication of
   multiple bouts of cholangitis, especially in patients
   with congenital ductal anatomic abnormalities.

PITFALLS

1. Ultrasound is 95-98% accurate in diagnosing gallbladder
   stones and very effective in detecting ductal
   dilatation, but only detects 10-50% of common duct
   stones.

2. Charcot's triad (biliary colic, chills and fever, and
   jaundice) is seen in only 70% of patients with
   ascending cholangitis. Twenty percent are never
   febrile and 25% are not jaundiced.

3. Painless obstructive jaundice is often considered a
   sign of malignant involvement of the biliary tract, but
   occasional patients with choledocholithiasis present
   with multiple stones and painless jaundice.

4. Blood cultures are positive in only 50% of patients
   with ascending cholangitis and may be positive for a
   different organism than in the bile culture.

SUGGESTED READINGS

Allen AF, Borody TJ, Bogliosi TF, et al: Rapid dissolution
   of gallstones in humans using methyl tertiarybutyl
   ether. Gastroenterology 88:122, 1985.
Berk JE, Meshkinpour H, Shapiro M, et al:
   Choledocholithiasis. In Berk J, et al (eds): Bockus
   Gastroenterology, ed. 4. Philadelphia, WB Saunders,
   1985, pp 3693-3705.
Gogel HK, Runyon BA, Volpicelli NA, et al: Acute
   suppurative obstruction cholangitis due to stones.
   Treatment by urgent endoscopic sphincterotomy. Gastro
   Endosc 33:210, 1987.
Kalser MH, Block MA: Cholangitis. In Berk J, et al (eds):
   Bockus Gastroenterology, ed. 4. Philadelphia, WB
   Saunders, 1985, pp 3717-3724

Palmer KR, Hofmann AF: Intraductal mono-octanoin for
    the direct dissolution of bile duct stones: Experience
    in 343 patients.   Gut 27:196, 1986.
Patwardhan RV, Smith OJ, Farmelant MH: Serum transaminase
    levels and cholescintigraphic abnormalities in acute
    biliary tract obstruction.   Arch Int Med 147:1249,
    1987.
Thompson JE, Tompkins RK, Lonm WP: Factors in the
    management of acute cholangitis.   Ann Surg 195:137,
    1982.

CASE 36: ACUTE LOWER GI BLEEDING IN A 78-YEAR-OLD WOMAN

A 78-year-old woman presents to the emergency room with a
history of rectal bleeding for the past several hours. She
initially felt the urge to have a bowel movement but passed
only red blood and clots with no stool. She subsequently
has had 4 more bloody movements and now complains of
lightheadedness and dizziness. She denies any abdominal
pain. There is no history of gastrointestinal bleeding or
other disorders. She takes occasional aspirins and is
currently taking a diuretic for mild hypertension. There
has been no change in her bowel habits or weight. Her
pulse is 100 supine and 128 sitting. Her blood pressure is
90/56 supine and 80/40 sitting. Cardiac examination
reveals a tachycardia and a grade III/VI systolic ejection
murmur at the aortic area. The abdomen is soft and
nontender with no masses or organomegaly. Bowel sounds are
normal. Rectal examination reveals bright red blood with
no stool. A nasogastric tube was passed and clear bile
stained fluid was aspirated. A sigmoidoscopy performed in
the emergency room was unhelpful as red blood was seen on
entering the rectum and obscured further evaluation.
Initial laboratory data reveals a hemoglobin of 11.8 g% and
normal coagulation studies.

TECHNETIUM SCAN CLUE

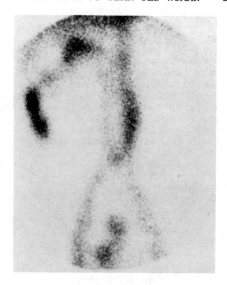

QUESTIONS

1. What is your differential diagnosis based upon the history and physical examination?

2. What diagnostic studies should be done immediately and over the next 24-48 hours to establish the etiology of the bleeding?

3. Why do diverticula bleed and what nonsurgical strategy can be used to stop the hemorrhage?

4. What are the angiographic findings in angiodysplasia?

5. What nonsurgical measures should be considered for treatment of arteriovenous malformation (AVM)-induced bleeding.

ANSWERS

1. a. Anal pathology, such as hemorrhoids, could result in painless rectal bleeding, but one would not expect evidence of hemodynamic instability.
    b. Ischemic bowel disease could be considered, particularly in this elderly patient, but the clinical picture usually resembles a colitis process. This patient had no abdominal pain and the rectal discharge contained no stool.
    c. Late onset inflammatory bowel disease could present with rectal bleeding, but the absence of diarrhea, pain or fever makes this possibility less likely.
    d. Painless rectal bleeding in the elderly suggests diverticular bleeding, AVM's of the right colon or neoplasm.

2. a. As with any bleeding patient the initial priority should be the restoration of hemodynamic stability.
    b. A nasogastric tube should be inserted to rule out the possibility of upper gastrointestinal bleeding. (There was no blood in the gastric aspirate.) The normal bowel sounds would tend to reduce this likelihood, since a considerable degree of bleeding, an excellent stimulus for peristalsis, would be necessary to result in red rectal bleeding from an upper GI site.
    c. Most lower gastrointestinal bleeding (75-80%) spontaneously stops and elective colonoscopy can then be performed. Colonoscopy during an active bleed may be very difficult due to blood obscuring the examination. Sigmoidoscopy, however, should be done early to at least try to evaluate the rectum in order to rule out hemorrhoidal bleeding, ulcerative colitis, rectal ulcers or ischemic colitis. The sigmoidoscopy in this patient showed normal mucosa with blood coming from "above."
    d. If the bleeding persists a technetium-99m sulphur colloid scan or tagged red blood cell study may be useful in localizing the general area of bleeding. Arteriography may then be used to more precisely determine the source of the bleeding. This technetium scan shows isotope extravasation in the region of the ascending colon, suggestive of bleeding from either diverticular disease or angiodysplasia (see Clue).

3. Twenty to 50% of the population over 50 years of age have diverticula, but bleeding occurs in only 3-5% of these patients. Hemorrhage results from a localized inflammatory reaction in a single diverticulum which erodes into a feeding vessel, usually with no evidence

of clinical diverticulitis. Seventy percent of diverticular bleeds arise from diverticula in the right colon despite the predominance in distribution of diverticula in the sigmoid colon. Eighty percent of diverticular bleeds stop spontaneously. Those that do not may be controlled at arteriography with intra-arterial infusion of vasopressin. If the bleeding cannot be controlled the surgeon can use the arteriographic findings to limit the extent of the segmental colonic resection.

4. Angiography demonstrates an early filling (arterial phase) vascular tuft, with a persistent blush of this collection of vessels and an early appearing prominent draining vein. If the lesion is bleeding at a rate greater than 0.5 to 1.0 ml/minute, dye extravasation into the lumen of the bowel may also be seen. Vasopressin infusion rarely will establish long-term control of active angiodysplastic bleeding. This patient demonstrated the typical angiographic features of cecal angiodysplasias.

5. Angiodysplasia or AVM's are irregular submucosal clusters of arterial, venous and capillary vessels, most commonly seen in the cecum and ascending colon, although they can occur anywhere in the gastrointestinal tract. They account for approximately 10-25% of major colonic hemorrhage, more often in the elderly, and are also a common cause of chronic recurrent slow bleeding. The lesions are frequently multiple and may be associated with aortic stenosis (10-15%). The bleeding is painless and may either be manifested as chronic heme-positive stools, melena or massive acute red rectal bleeding. Colonoscopy offers the advantage of identification and perhaps thermal control of the lesions with the heater probe or bicap probe, but this is difficult during the hemorrhage and it may not be clear as to which AVM has bled if the study is done later. Arteriography is useful in ascertaining the particular bleeding lesion if extravasation is seen; however, because of the nature of the vascular lesion, vasopressin infusion rarely provides long-term control and surgical resection is usually required for those with major hemorrhage or chronic bleeding. Embolization therapy with Gelfoam may be attempted in the poor surgical candidate but is risky because of the possibility of causing bowel infarction. Bleeding stopped in this patient and no surgery was performed. Three weeks later this patient bled again and a right hemicolectomy was performed.

PEARLS

1. Although diverticular bleeding in most patients stops
    spontaneously, 20-25% will rebleed shortly thereafter
    but others will have no recurrences. Therefore,
    surgery should be considered for those patients who
    have had multiple episodes of diverticular bleeding.

2. A normal BUN during an episode of red rectal bleeding
    strongly suggests a lower GI site since blood in the
    small bowel results in protein absorption and an
    increased BUN.

3. It is unusual for bleeding from a colonic polyp to be
    of sufficient magnitude to cause hemodynamic
    instability. Polyps bleed because they outgrow their
    blood supply, thus the lessened likelihood of erosion
    into a major blood vessel.

4. Recurrent bleeding from AVM's associated with aortic
    stenosis may cease after aortic valve replacement.
    Elective surgery for angiodysplasias should be
    postponed until after valve replacement to determine
    whether bleeding recurs.

5. Colonoscopy can be performed during an episode of
    colonic bleeding if a colonic lavage with an
    electrolyte solution (Golytely, Colyte) is administered
    and the hemodynamic status is monitored carefully. The
    advantage of this approach is that the causative AVM or
    diverticulum can be identified with greater confidence.

PITFALLS

1. Barium studies have no role in the evaluation of major
    lower gastrointestinal bleeding since AVM's cannot be
    seen and the barium will make subsequent angiography or
    colonoscopy impossible until the barium can be cleared
    from the colon.

2. Since angiodysplasia is a common finding in the
    elderly, one cannot definitively ascribe bleeding to
    these lesions unless extravasation into the bowel lumen
    is seen at angiography or bleeding is actually seen
    colonoscopically. Surgery should not be performed
    because of the presence of AVM's which have not been
    identified as the bleeding source.

3. If the source of red rectal bleeding is in doubt, upper endoscopy should be performed to rule out a proximal source since 15% of presumed "lower" gastrointestinal bleeding turns out to be secondary to peptic ulcer disease.

4. Red rectal bleeding may arise from the upper gastrointestinal tract if bowel transit is rapid enough and melena may arise from sites as distal as the ascending colon if transit time is sufficiently slow, therefore the color of the stool cannot always distinguish between upper and lower gastrointestinal bleeding.

SUGGESTED READINGS

Cappell MS, Lebwohl O: Cessation of recurrent bleeding from gastrointestinal angiodysplasia after aortic valve replacement. Ann Int Med 105:54, 1986.

Isselbacher KJ, Richter JM: Hematemesis, melena and hematochezia. In Braunwald E, et al (eds): Harrison's Principles of Internal Medicine, ed. 11. New York, McGraw Hill, 1987, pp 180-183.

Koval G, Benner KG, Rosch J, et al: Aggressive angiographic diagnosis in acute lower gastrointestinal hemorrhage. Dig Dis Sci 32:248, 1987.

Meyer CT, Troncale FJ, Galloway S, et al: Arteriovenous malformations of the bowel: An analysis of 22 cases and a review of the literature. Medicine 60:36, 1981.

Richter JM, Hedberg SE, Athanasoulis CA, et al: Angiodysplasia: Clinical presentation and colonoscopic diagnosis. Dig Dis Sci 29:481, 1984.

Steer ML, Silen W: Diagnostic procedures in gastrointestinal hemorrhage. N Engl J Med 309:646, 1983.

Thompson NW: Vascular ectasias and colonic diverticula: Common causes of lower gastrointestinal hemorrhage in the aged. In Fiddian-Green RG, Turcotte JG (eds): Gastrointestinal Hemorrhage. New York, Grune & Stratton, 1980, pp 375-388.

CASE 37: ACUTE UPPER GI BLEEDING IN AN ALCOHOLIC

A 48-year-old accountant presents to the emergency room
with the history of having felt well until 2 hours
previously when he became nauseous and subsequently
vomited a large amount of red blood and clots. He has
since had 2 more episodes of similar hematemesis. He
denies any abdominal pain. There is no past history of
gastrointestinal bleeding or peptic ulcer disease. The
patient admits to a long history of heavy alcohol use and
cigarette smoking. He takes no medications. His blood
pressure is 90/40 mm Hg and his pulse is 120/min. His
sclera are icteric and there are spider angiomas on the
chest. The liver measures 14 cm in the midclavicular line
and the spleen is palpable 3 cm below the left costal
margin. The abdominal examination reveals moderate
distension, shifting dullness and hyperactive bowel sounds.

CLUE

Hgb/Hct 9.6/28.4, platelet count 92,000; prothrombin time
C10.6/T15.8 sec, bilirubin 3.8, alkaline phosphatase 120,
AST (SGOT) 264, ALT (SGPT) 112, total protein 7.8, albumin
2.9, cholesterol 100.

QUESTIONS

1. What is your differential diagnosis at this point?

2. Why is early endoscopy important in this patient?

3. What therapeutic measures should be considered?

4. What is the mortality rate for the 1st episode of hemorrhage from esophageal varices?

5. How common is variceal bleeding in cirrhosis and what causes the varices to bleed?

6. What is the success rate of esophageal variceal sclerotherapy and what are the complications?

7. Do portal-systemic shunts improve survival from variceal hemorrhage?

8. What long-term pharmacologic measures have been used in an effort to prevent rebleeding from varices?

ANSWERS

1. This patient has multiple stigmata of chronic liver
    disease, probably but not definitely of alcoholic
    origin (15% of patients with an alcoholic history are
    found to have liver disease of some other cause). The
    ascites and splenomegaly suggest the presence of
    cirrhosis and portal hypertension. Although esophageal
    varices are likely in this patient, varices are the
    cause of only 50% of upper gastrointestinal bleeding in
    the cirrhotic patient. Chronic gastritis is common in
    portal hypertension, probably due to mucosal congestion
    as well as the toxic effects of alcohol. Peptic ulcer
    disease, esophagitis and Mallory-Weiss tears are also
    common in this patient population.

2. After hemodynamic stabilization and attempts to control
    the coagulopathy with fresh frozen plasma and vitamin
    K, endoscopy is required to distinguish between
    esophageal varices and other causes for upper GI
    bleeding. Varices require different treatment
    considerations than bleeding from a Mallory-Weiss tear,
    esophagitis or peptic ulcer disease. This patient was
    found to be bleeding from large varices in the distal
    esophagus.

3. Sclerotherapy during the bleeding may be successful in
    stopping or reducing the blood loss, thus decreasing
    the hemodynamic risks and need for transfusions. If
    technical problems preclude the procedure, intravenous
    pitressin can be used to reduce cardiac output and
    portal venous return, thus lowering portal pressure.
    The infusion should begin with 0.4 units/minute and can
    be gradually increased every several hours to a maximum
    of 1 unit/minute. This approach may be contraindicated
    if the patient has coronary artery disease since
    coronary arterial filling is diminished and angina or
    other cardiac problems may be induced. Some groups
    advise coadministration of sublingual nitroglycerin to
    reduce the adverse cardiac effects. If the patient
    fails to respond to these measures, a
    Sengstaken-Blakemore tube may be required to tamponade
    the varices, although the frequency of complications
    related to the device rises to approximately 50% after
    72 hours of inflation. If brisk hemorrhage fails to
    subside, emergency portacaval shunt can be considered,
    but the mortality rate is approximately 50%.

4. The mortality rate for the 1st admission with variceal
    bleeding is 25-50%. The mortality varies with the

etiology of the varices. Patients with extrahepatic portal or splenic vein thrombosis and normal liver function tolerate bleeding fairly well, as do patients with hepatic schistosomiasis who have well-preserved liver function. Alcoholic cirrhotics, especially those with significant hepatic parenchymal dysfunction do poorly. The risk of rebleeding and death is highest in the 1st few days after the 1st bleed. One-third of those who survive the initial hemorrhage rebleed within the next 6 weeks. The 1-year survival after the initial bleed is only 35-50%.

5. Only 20-40% of all patients with alcoholic cirrhosis ever bleed from esophageal varices. This relatively low incidence coupled with the high morbidity and mortality of portal-systemic shunt procedures accounts for the lack of utility for prophylactic shunting in patients with varices who have never bleed. Bleeding, when it occurs, is due to a single pinhole eruption of a varix. Variceal size, not the height of portal pressure, is felt to correlate best with the likelihood of bleeding. Although bleeding is rare when portal pressures are less than 12 mm Hg, there is no direct correlation between the height of portal pressures greater than 12 mm Hg and variceal bleeding. Erosion of varices from peptic reflux is probably not a major pathophysiologic mechanism since esophageal pH probe monitoring has not shown an increased incidence of reflux in patients with variceal bleeding.

6. Variceal sclerotherapy is accomplished by injection of a sclerosing agent such as sodium tetradecyl, sodium morrhuate, polidocanol or ethanolamine oleate directly into (intravariceal) or adjacent to the varix (paravariceal), or a combination of both techniques. Acutely, there is an inflammatory reaction in the vessel that causes thrombosis. A fibrotic reaction occurs later. Successful control of acute bleeding is achieved in 90% of patients but sclerotherapy must be repeated periodically until all varices are treated. Rebleeding occurs in 20-60% in various series. There is a less than 1% mortality rate with sclerotherapy and a 10-15% complication rate, including esophageal ulcerations, stricture or perforation, fever, pneumonitis, mediastinitis and pleural effusions. Prophylactic sclerotherapy (performed in patients with varices who have not bled) has no proven clinical benefit.

7. Although extremely effective in preventing rebleeding
    if the patient survives the surgery, overall survival
    is unchanged after portal-sytemic shunts. The patients
    die from other complications of end-stage liver
    disease, such as hepatic encephalopathy, hepatic
    failure or HRS. Therefore, nonsurgical alternatives
    such as medical therapy and sclerotherapy have received
    much attention. No difference in long-term survival
    has been reported in groups treated with sclerotherapy
    as compared to surgery.

8. Propranolol, a nonselective beta blocker, has been
    shown to lower both portal pressure and cardiac output
    Although initially reported to be highly successful in
    preventing rebleeding from esophageal varices,
    subsequent studies have shown less convincing benefit.
    Another problem with beta blockade is that if the
    patient does rebleed he may be unable to mount a
    physiologic increase in heart rate to maintain his
    cardiac output. A recent study showed a lower
    incidence of death and 1st bleeding in patients found
    to have esophageal varices who were treated with
    prophylactic propranolol. This also warrants further
    investigation.

PEARLS

1. All of the sequellae of portal hypertension such as
    variceal bleeding, ascites, etc., can occur with acute
    reversible alcoholic hepatitis and does not necessarily
    indicate the presence of cirrhosis.

2. Cessation of alcoholic intake has been shown to
    decrease portal hypertension in patients with "early"
    cirrhosis. This is not true for patients with
    end-stage cirrhosis.

3. Bleeding from esophageal varices usually occurs in the
    distal esophagus, within 1.5 cm of the esophagogastric
    junction. Approximately 10% of variceal bleeding is
    from gastric varices. These varices are poorly treated
    with sclerotherapy as the early rebleeding rate
    approaches 100%.

4. Although studies have shown no difference in long-term
    survival between groups treated with sclerotherapy or
    portal-systemic shunts, early studies suggested a lower
    cost associated with variceal sclerotherapy. However,
    when these patients are followed for a longer period o

time, the higher rebleeding rate in the sclerotherapy group, requiring more hospital readmissions and need for multiple transfusions, may eventually make the total medical care costs of both groups about the same.

5. Patients who had undergone portacaval shunts were initially viewed as unacceptable for liver transplant because of the increased technical problems. Transplant teams currently view previously shunted patients with less concern.

PITFALLS

1. The Sengstaken-Blakemore tube has no esophageal aspiration port, thus leading to accumulations of pharyngeal secretions above the inflated esophageal or gastric balloon and subsequent aspiration. A nasogastric tube should be positioned above the balloons for suction purposes. Alternatively, there is a variant of the Sengstaken-Blakemore tube which includes a suction port above the balloons. If a patient becomes acutely cyanotic while the balloons are inflated, the gastric balloon may have ruptured, allowing the esophageal balloon to pull up and occlude the larynx, necessitating immediate decompression of the balloon. If this occurs, the tube should be cut with a scissors to decompress the balloons. When inserting the tube, extreme care must be taken to insure proper placement since inflation of the gastric balloon in the esophagus can be catastrophic.

2. Mortality is highest in the 1st several days after the initial bleed from esophageal varices, therefore studies comparing efficacies of 1 modality of treatment with others must be critically evaluated for the "starting point" of the therapy. If, for example, the modality in question is initiated only in patients stable 2 weeks after the initial bleed, the highest mortality group has already been selected out.

3. Reduce saline and total fluid administration once bleeding has stopped since overly aggressive replacement usually leads to ascites and can also raise the portal pressure.

4. Patients with poor liver function frequently show signs of hepatic encephalopathy during a major hemorrhage. Lactulose should be started as soon as bleeding stops,

not only to reduce the serum NH3 but also to eliminate the residual blood (and its protein content) from the gut.

5. Do not forget that inadequate blood replacement is the most common preventable cause of death in all patients with gastrointestinal bleeding. A patient may require 2 units given simultaneously and perhaps under pressure in order to keep up with brisk blood loss.

SUGGESTED READINGS

Burroughs AK, Jenkins WJ, Sherlock S, et al: Controlled trial of propranolol for the prevention of recurrent variceal hemorrhage in patients with cirrhosis. N Engl J Med 309:1539, 1983.

Cello JP, Grendell JH, Cross RA, et al: Endoscopic sclerotherapy versus portacaval shunt in patients with severe cirrhosis and acute variceal hemorrhage. Long term follow-up. N Engl J Med 316:11, 1987.

Chojkier M, Conn HO: Esophageal tamponade in the treatment of bleeding varices. Dig Dis Sci 25:267, 1980.

Pasal JP, Cales P, and a multicenter study group: Propranolol in the prevention of 1st upper gastrointestinal tract hemorrhage in patients with cirrhosis of the liver and esophageal varices. N Engl J Med 317;856, 1987.

Santangelo WC, Dueno MI, Estes BL, et al: Prophylactic sclerotherapy of large esophageal varices. N Engl J Med 318:814, 1988.

Schuman BM, Beckman JW, Tedesco FJ, et al: Complications of endoscopic injection sclerotherapy: A review. Am J Gastroenterol 82:823, 1987.

Sorensen TIA: Sclerotherapy after 1st variceal hemorrhage in cirrhosis. A randomized multicenter trial--The Copenhagen esophageal varices sclerotherapy project. N Engl J Med 311:1594, 1984.

Sutton FM: Upper gastrointestinal bleeding in patients with esophageal varices: What is the most common source? Am J Med 83:273, 1987.

Terblanche J, Bornman PC, Kahn D, et al: The management of acute variceal bleeding. In Popper H, Schaffner F (eds): Progress in Liver Diseases, vol. 8. New York, Grune & Stratton, 1986, pp 541-555.

Westaby D, Williams R: Portal hypertension. In Berk JE (ed): Bockus Gastroenterology, ed. 4. Philadelphia, WB Saunders, 1985, pp 3062-3082.

CASE 38: A JAUNDICED INTRAVENOUS DRUG USER

A 38-year-old man comes to your office complaining of
decreased appetite, a 10-pound weight loss, weakness and
low grade fevers for several weeks. He is an intravenous
drug user with no history of hepatitis and drinks several
beers per day.   He has not been on any prescribed
medications. Physical examination reveals normal vital
signs.   His sclera are slightly icteric. The skin appears
normal, there are no spider angioma or other stigmata of
chronic liver disease. The liver measures 14 cm in span in
the right midclavicular line and is mildly tender to
palpation. The spleen is not palpable. There is no
ascites. Laboratory evaluation reveals a bilirubin of 2.9
mg%, AST (SGOT) 245 units, ALT (SGPT) 320 units, alkaline
phosphatase 80 units, total protein 7.5g% and albumin
4.2g%. An ultrasound study shows a normal pancreas and
gallbladder.

CLUE

Hepatitis viral serology reveals a positive HBsAg, negative anti-HBs, and negative anti-HAV.

QUESTIONS

1. How can you determine if this is acute or chronic hepatitis B disease?

2. Should this patient have a liver biopsy? Why?

3. The patient asks whether he is infectious to others. What study will help determine his infectivity?

4. If a patient with chronic active hepatitis B experiences an acute exacerbation, what etiology should you consider?

5. What lethal complication, other than those resulting from the severity of the liver disease (encephalopathy, portal hypertension, ascites), occurs in patients with chronic hepatitis B disease?

6. Distinguish between hepatitis B and non-A non-B (NANB) in respect to:
   a. Incubation period.

   b. Percentage of patients who progress to a chronic phase.

   c. Frequency after blood transfusion.

ANSWERS

1.   The HB core antibody (anti-HBc) is very helpful in
     distinguishing acute from chronic disease. IgM
     anti-HBc appears early after acute hepatitis B, usually
     persists for 4-6 months and is subsequently replaced by
     IgG anti-HBc, which can be detected for years after the
     primary infection. This patient had a positive IgG
     anti-HBc suggesting that his hepatitis B infection is
     chronic.

2.   The liver biopsy can serve to distinguish between
     chronic persistent hepatitis (portal inflammation
     without piecemeal necrosis or bridging), chronic active
     hepatitis (piecemeal necrosis, which may be associated
     with inflammatory bridging between portal spaces) and
     cirrhosis. In this case, chronic persistent hepatitis
     is unlikely because of the jaundice, so that the biopsy
     can be used to "stage" the severity of the hepatitis
     and exclude other disorders, such as alcoholic and
     granulomatous hepatitis. This patient's biopsy showed
     evidence of chronic active hepatitis with transition to
     cirrhosis.

3.   The hepatitis E antigen (HBeAg), which was positive in
     this patient, is an indication of viral replication and
     the presence of intact virus in the blood. This is
     usually a sign of active liver disease. The presence
     of hepatitis B DNA polymerase in the serum would
     provide similar information. The conversion of HBeAg
     to anti-HBe (approximately 10% per year in patients
     with chronic hepatitis), reflects resolution of
     hepatitis B virus replication.

4.   A subsequent infection with delta virus should be
     considered. This is a defective RNA virus which
     requires the presence of hepatitis B virus to survive.
     A patient may be coinfected with delta virus at the
     time of the initial infection with hepatitis B, which
     can lead to a fulminant hepatitis or acquire the virus
     as a superinfection, which often results in an
     exacerbation of the hepatitis B disease. Forty percent
     of the latter patients will progress to cirrhosis.
     Although there is no known therapy for delta or
     hepatitis B virus, hepatitis B vaccine provides
     protection against both viruses.

5.   Hepatoma is associated with chronic hepatitis B
     disease, often occurring in chronic carriers. There
     are an estimated 200 million such patients in the

world, many of whom live in 3rd world countries and
have harbored the virus from birth, thus leading to
250,000 hepatomas diagnosed each year and establishing
hepatomas as 1 of the most common solid tumors.

6. a. NANB hepatitis has an incubation period averaging 7
    weeks (2-26 weeks), while hepatitis B is approximately
    2-6 months.
    b. Approximately 10% of patients with hepatitis B
    progress to chronic hepatitis (more than 6 months
    duration of inflammatory change), while 30% of patients
    with NANB hepatitis enter a chronic phase. Although
    this is often a subclinical process, approximately 10%
    of these patients progress to postnecrotic cirrhosis.
    c. NANB hepatitis has replaced hepatitis B as the
    primary cause of post-transfusion hepatitis.

PEARLS

1. Patients with chronic hepatitis B disease should be
    screened with interval alpha-fetoprotein and hepatic
    ultrasound for the early detection of hepatoma.

2. Survival in chronic hepatitis B is directly related to
    the histologic changes. The 5-year survival for
    chronic persistent hepatitis is 97%, for chronic active
    hepatitis without cirrhosis it is 86% and in patients
    with chronic active hepatitis with cirrhosis it is 55%.

3. An unvaccinated person who has a percutaneous exposure
    to serum from a known HBsAg positive source should
    receive both hepatitis B immune globulin and hepatitis
    B vaccination. The likelihood of developing hepatitis
    B following a needle stick from a known hepatitis B
    "donor" is approximately 9%, which can be significantly
    reduced with active and passive immunization.

4. The incidence of post-transfusion NANB hepatitis is
    markedly lowered by using blood only from volunteer
    donors or by screening transfused blood with serum
    glutamic pyruvic transaminase (SGPT ALT) levels and
    discarding all blood with elevated values.

5. The likelihood of developing chronic hepatitis B
    disease is much greater in childhood. Almost all
    children contracting the infection during the 1st few
    months of life progress to chronic infection and are at
    the highest risk of developing hepatoma.

PITFALLS

1. There is no effective therapy for hepatitis B disease.
    Corticosteroids are associated with serologic evidence
    of enhanced viral replication, more frequent
    complications and a higher mortality rate.
    Azathioprine, vidarafine (ARA-A), interferon and
    acyclovir have all failed to change the course of the
    disease, but efforts to develop an antiviral therapy
    are continuing.

2. Seroconversion from positive HBeAg to positive anti-HBe
    does not necessarily imply permanent remission.
    Approximately 1/3 of patients who enter this
    "nonreplicative" phase will then revert back to HBeAg
    positivity within 1 year and reactivate their
    disease.

3. The duration of effective immunity following hepatitis
    B vaccination is presently unclear. A recent study
    showed 38% of hospital employees to have low antibody
    levels 3 years after the vaccination, although these
    individuals may still have some degree of immunity. It
    is possible that revaccination will be required for
    many healthy adults.

4. HBsAg may persist in the liver after it has been lost
    in the serum. Therefore, although rare, a negative
    HBsAg in the serum of a patient with chronic hepatitis
    does not absolutely rule out hepatitis B as the cause.

SUGGESTED READINGS

Bisceglie AM, Rustgi VK, Hoofnagle JH, et al:
    Hepatocellular carcinoma. Ann Int Med 108:390, 1988.
Boyer JL, Miller DJ: Chronic hepatitis. In Schiff L,
    Schiff ER (eds): Diseases of the Liver, ed. 6.
    Philadelphia, JB Lippincott, 1987, pp 687-723.
Cock KM, Govindarajan S, Chin KP, et al: Delta Hepatitis
    in the Los Angeles Area: A report of 126 cases. Ann
    Int Med 105:108, 1986.
Hoofnagle JH, Shafritz DA, Popper H: Chronic type B
    hepatitis and the "healthy" HBsAg carrier state.
    Hepatology 7:758, 1987.
Horowitz MM, Ershler WB, McKinney WP, et al: Duration of
    immunity after hepatitis B vaccination: Efficacy of
    low-dose booster vaccine. Ann Int Med 108:185, 1988.

Liaw Y-F, Tai DI, Chu CM, et al: Early detection of
    hepatocellular carcinoma in patients with chronic type
    B hepatitis. Gastroenterology 90:263, 1987.
Schiff E: Immunoprophylaxis of viral hepatitis: A
    practical guide. Am J Gastroenterol 82:287, 1987.

CASE 39: MASSIVE SMALL BOWEL RESECTION

A 79-year-old man with severe coronary artery disease,
chronic atrial fibrillation and congestive heart failure
develops acute diffuse abdominal pain. There has been no
nausea or vomiting. Present medications include nitrates,
calcium blockers, diuretics and digoxin. His termperature
is 99.6 F, the pulse is 110/min and irregular and the blood
pressure is 110/60. Bowel sounds are hyperactive and mild
periumbilical tenderness is present without peritoneal
signs. There are no masses or abdominal bruits.
Laboratory studies show the following: white blood count
is 26,800 with 82% polys, 14% bands and 4% lymphs;
hemoglobin 13.6 g%, hematocrit 40.6%, amylase 92 units
(normal to 100 units). An obstruction series reveals a
nonspecific gas pattern in the small bowel and no evidence
of free intra-abdominal air.

ANGIOGRAPHIC CLUE

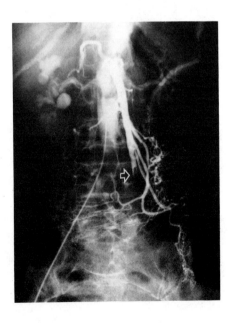

QUESTIONS

1. What diagnoses would you consider?

2. This patient will be left with a "short bowel" syndrome. What are other causes can you list for this condition?

3. What factors are important in determining how a patient with a massive small bowel resection survives the postoperative period?

4. What happens to gastric acid secretion after extensive bowel resection?

5. What are the major clinical and laboratory features of the short bowel syndrome?

6. What postoperative and chronic therapy would you outline for this patient?

ANSWERS

1. Common causes of abdominal pain, such as peptic ulcer
   disease, pancreatitis, bowel obstruction with
   perforation, appendicitis and biliary tract disease,
   were all possible, but the cardiac problems present in
   this patient should seriously suggest the possibility
   of mesenteric ischemia. This could result from
   nonocclusive mechanisms secondary to a period of
   decreased cardiac output in association with a
   diminished blood volume (diuretic therapy) and
   increased peripheral resistance (digitalis effect). A
   thrombosis or embolic occlusion of a mesenteric vessel
   should also be considered. An arteriogram was
   performed, and revealed an embolus of the superior
   mesenteric artery (see Clue). An embolectomy was
   urgently performed but sufficient gut ischemia had
   occurred to require a resection of approximately 80% of
   the proximal and mid small bowel. The proximal jejunum
   was anastomosed to the distal ileum.

2. Most causes of short bowel syndrome occur from massive
   resection for acute vascular incidents, as in this
   patient. Multiple intestinal resections due to
   complications of Crohn's disease is another common
   cause. The jejunoileal bypass procedures for obesity
   (rarely performed now), small bowel volvulus, trauma,
   necrotizing enterocolitis and congenital short bowel
   are additional causes.

3. Forty to 50% of the small bowel can be removed without
   impairment to normal nutrition, depending on what
   segment of small bowel is removed, the presence of the
   ileocecal valve, and the functional integrity of the
   remaining small bowel. The proximal small bowel is
   primarily responsible for water, electrolyte and
   nutrient absorption, while the ileum is important for
   bile salt and vitamin B-12 absorption. Loss of the
   jejunum is better tolerated than loss of the duodenum
   or terminal ileum. Absence of the ileocecal valve
   leads to bacterial contamination of the small bowel
   with colonic anaerobic flora, resulting in
   deconjugation of bile salts and bacterial utilization
   of vitamin B-12. The colon serves primarily for water
   absorption and therefore influences the eventual volume
   of diarrhea. If the remaining small bowel is healthy
   (which it may not be in Crohn's disease), "intestinal
   adaptation" occurs, characterized by cellular
   hyperplasia which increases the potential absorptive
   area, a process which takes place over many months.

4. Gastric acid hypersecretion is common in the early
    postoperative period. Gastrin levels are increased
    after surgery due to decreased gastrin catabolism
    resulting from the loss of small bowel surface area as
    well as the presence of increased gastrin inhibitors
    such as secretin, cholecystokinin (CCK), vasoactive
    intestinal polypeptide (VIP) and gastric inhibitory
    polypeptide (GIP). The resulting hyperacidity may lead
    to inactivation of pancreatic enzymes, deconjugation of
    bile salts and small bowel injury, events similar to
    those encountered in the Zollinger-Ellison syndrome and
    contribute to the diarrhea which occurs after extensive
    small bowel resection. Histamine-2 receptor
    antagonists should be given in the immediate
    postoperative period to control the hyperacidity. The
    process is self-limited and subsides within several
    weeks or months.

5. Watery diarrhea, steatorrhea, acidosis and electrolyte
    abnormalities are the major features of the short bowel
    syndrome. The magnitude of the abnormalities depends
    on the site and extent of bowel resection. The
    malabsorption syndrome is similar to that encountered
    in severe sprue, with weight loss, fatigue,
    hypocalcemia, vitamin D deficiency and metabolic bone
    disease. Vitamin B-12, iron and folate deficiencies
    occur.

    Failure to complex oxalate with luminal calcium leads
    to the formation of calcium oxalate renal stones and
    failure to maintain a bile acid pool may result in
    cholesterol gallstones.

6. Maintenance of fluid and electrolyte balance,
    prevention of hypersecretion of acid with
    H2-antagonists and total parenteral nutrition (TPN) are
    the cornerstones of the immediate postoperative
    therapy. Enteral nutrition should be added as soon as
    possible to provide trophic stimuli to the remaining
    small bowel. Elemental feedings through a nasogastric
    tube can satisfy this need. When oral feedings are
    begun, it may be necessary to use multiple small
    feedings utilizing medium chain triglycerides for at
    least 30% of the fat source, and a low lactose and
    oxalate diet. Codeine, diphenoxylate, loperamide and
    anticholinergic agents may be useful in decreasing
    diarrhea. Antibiotics should be considered if small
    bowel bacterial overgrowth secondary to loss of the
    ileocecal valve occurs. Pancreatic enzymes can be
    helpful if a proximal resection has been performed,

since stimulation with cholecystokinin may be deficient. If adequate oral nutrition cannot be achieved, home TPN can be offered on a temporary basis (until intestinal adaptation occurs) or permanently. Occasional success has been reported with antiperistaltic small bowel loop reversals to slow transit and improve absorption.

PEARLS

1. There may be difficulty in establishing whether resection margins are viable in patients with mesenteric ischemia, thus the need to consider a "2nd look" procedure in 24-48 hours to establish the circulatory status of the anastomosis in selected patients.

2. If the colon is intact, fluid and electrolyte losses are not excessive, unless the fluid load exceeds the colon's reserve capacity of approximately 5 liters/day. Therefore, proximal resection results in little diarrhea because the ileum is capable of reabsorbing the increased fluid and electrolyte load and the remaining excess is absorbed by the colon. If both the ileum and the colon are resected, the remaining bowel cannot sufficiently concentrate luminal contents, leading to severe isotonic water and salt loss, resulting in dehydration, hypokalemia and hypomagnesemia, the so-called end-jejunostomy syndrome.

3. When the jejunum alone is removed, the ileum takes over the absorptive functions and malabsorption is minimal, while ileal resections of only 100 cm cause steatorrhea. Resections up to 33% usually do not result in malnutrition and up to 50% can be tolerated without special aids. When resections exceed 75% of the bowel, nutrition cannot be maintained without special assistance.

4. If the patient has more than 60-80 cm of small bowel remaining, an oral diet of natural foods should be tried, with advice to take liquids 1 hour after solids because of the faster rate of gastric emptying after massive resections. Although a low fat diet with medium chain triglyceride feedings has been the classically described approach-to-the-short-bowel syndrome, there is sufficient disagreement in the literature regarding the adverse effects of fat on diarrhea that a trial of fat in the diet should be

considered.   Indeed, some workers feel that the
distribution of fat, carbohydrate and protein in the
diet may not be of significant importance in the
diarrhea and malabsorption stemming from massive bowel
resection.

PITFALLS

1. The cost of home TPN is in the range of $35,000-
    $50,000 yearly, not including catheter complications.

2. Although medium chain triglycerides are easier to
    absorb because micelle formation is not required, the
    taste is hard to disguise and patient compliance is
    poor.

3. Although the small bowel is described as being
    approximately 600 cm long, this measurement is obtained
    at the autopsy table. The small bowel contracts to
    approximately 350 cm in the living patient and surgeons
    who remove "several loops" may leave the patient with a
    short bowel syndrome.

4. Small bowel transplantation is an attractive
    consideration for patients with the short bowel
    syndrome who require permanent TPN. Unfortunately, the
    graft-versus-host process remains a major barrier,
    although there is considerable experimentation with
    cyclosporine, azathioprine, prednisone, antithymocyte
    globulin and monoclonal antibodies. At this time,
    there have been no long-term survivors of small bowel
    transplantation, but advances in preservation of
    cadaver grafts and control of graft-versus-host
    reactions suggest that clinical trials may be
    undertaken.

SUGGESTED READINGS

Jeejeebhoy KN: Therapy of the short-gut syndrome. Lancet
     2:1427, 1983.
Schraut WH: Current status of small-bowel transplantation.
     Gastroenterology 94:525, 1988.
Thompson JS, Rikkers LF: Surgical alternatives for the
     short bowel syndrome. Am J Gastroenterol 82:97, 1987.
Williams NS, Evans P, King RF: Gastric acid secretion and
     gastrin production in the short bowel syndrome. Gut
     26:914, 1985.

Woolf GM, Kurian R, Jeejeebhoy KN: Diet for patients with
    a short bowel: High fat or high carbohydrate?
    Gastroenterology 84:823, 1983.

CASE 40: ANAL PRURITUS AND DISCHARGE IN A YOUNG MAN

A 22-year-old male presents to your clinic with the
complaint of anal pruritus and mucus discharge of
approximately 2 weeks duration. He denies abdominal pain
and has normal bowel movements, although on 1 recent
occasion he noted a blood streak on the stool. There has
been no unusual travel history and he takes no medications,
although he had received antibiotic therapy several months
ago for a severe upper respiratory infection. The patient
is single and lives alone. Physical examination showed
normal vital signs and no abnormality of the chest or
abdomen. Inspection of the anus revealed no pathology but
the digital rectal examination was painful for the patient
and produced evidence of a mucopurulent discharge which was
positive for occult blood.   The CBC and urinalysis were
unremarkable.

CLUE

Sigmoidoscopy showed hyperemic and mildly friable mucosa with overlying mucopurulent exudate extending several centimeters above the dentate line. The mucosa was normal above this point to a distance of 20 cm.

QUESTIONS

1. What "lifestyle" information is required?

2. What is your differential diagnosis?

3. What additional studies are most important?

4. What therapy would you offer?

5. If this patient also had evidence of perirectal venereal warts (Condyloma acuminatum), what disease would he be more likely to develop?

ANSWERS

1. This patient has sigmoidoscopic evidence of a proctitis. It is important to determine whether the patient is homosexual since the spectrum of disease possibilities is significantly different from those encountered in heterosexual males. The rectal mucosa is more fragile than the vaginal mucosa so that trauma may lead to microscopic or macroscopic tears which permit invasion by a variety of bacterial and viral pathogens. This patient is homosexual and has had numerous partners in the previous several months.

2. Gonorrhea is the most common sexually transmitted disease (STD) in homosexual men and the rectum is the only site infected in 40%, most of whom are asymptomatic, although anorectal inflammation can occur. The most common symptoms are mucus on the stool and rectal discomfort. The inflammatory changes are limited to the anal canal and distal rectum but are not sufficiently characteristic to allow for a visual diagnosis. The diagnosis of anal gonorrhea remains a bacteriologic one.

   Although the primary chancre is the characteristic syphilitic lesion, it may be confused with other conditions such as rectal fissure, fistula or rectal ulcer. In addition, diffuse distal proctitis can occur.

   Herpetic infections are a common STD in homosexual men and should be strongly considered in the differential diagnosis of proctitis. Type II is the most common herpetic virus and is often associated with localized or grouped vesicular lesions in the perianal or genital area where the virus has locally invaded. An acute proctitis with mucopurulent exudate is also seen with this infection. Biopsies show nonspecific inflammatory changes and the diagnosis is usually based on the combination of characteristic skin lesions and proctitis. Acute and chronic phase complement fixation tests are helpful for confirming the diagnosis but require too much time to be clinically useful during the acute symptoms.

   Chlamydia-related proctitis has been recognized and is probably due to the nonlymphogranuloma venereum strain. The diagnosis is established by isolation of the organism and the proctitis usually responds to antibiotic therapy (oxytetracycline). The

lymphogranuloma venereum (LGV) strain of Chlamydia
trachomatis produces a reaction which varies from
proctitis to severe fistula and stricture formation.
The sigmoidoscopic findings may resemble Crohn's
disease and biopsies often show granulomas with giant
cells. Painful inguinal adenopathy may occur 4-6 weeks
after the exposure. The diagnosis can be established
by direct culture (about 50% sensitive) or by serologic
techniques (somewhat insensitive and may be associated
with false-positive reactions).

3. A rectal culture should be obtained, either through the
    sigmoidoscope or as a rectal swab, and plated directly
    onto a Thayer-Martin medium to evaluate for gonorrhea,
    and another sample should be taken for Chlamydia
    trachomatis. A Gram stain of the rectal smear should
    also be performed but will miss 50% of gonorrhea
    patients. Even though there is no apparent chancre in
    this patient, a serology for syphilis should be
    obtained. The culture was positive for gonorrhea in
    this patient. HIV infection is increasing in the
    population attending sexually transmitted disease (STD)
    clinics and testing should be considered if there are
    features to suggest its presence.

4. Single dose intramuscular procaine penicillin G plus 1
    g oral probenecid is effective for both anorectal and
    pharyngeal gonorrhea as well as syphilis in the
    prechancre stage. An oral ampicillin program of 3.5 g
    plus 1 g of oral probenicid is also effective against
    anorectal gonorrhea but appears to be less useful for
    pharyngeal infections.

5. Squamous cell cancer of the anus is more common in
    homosexual men and appears to be related to the
    presence of genital warts. Seropositivity for herpes
    simplex 2 or Chlamydia trachomatis infections also
    appears to be a risk factor for anal cancer. Rectal
    lymphoma also occurs more frequently in homosexual men.

PEARLS

1. Salmonella, Shigella and Campylobacter infections can
    be sexually transmitted. Less severe enteric symptoms
    (diarrhea, crampy pain or bloating) in homosexual males
    should also suggest the possibility of giardiasis or
    amebiasis.

2. Pharyngeal gonorrhea is usually asymptomatic (or results in a mild pharyngitis) in homosexual males but can be detected by appropriate throat cultures.

3. If proctitis extends beyond 10-15 cm, consider Campylobacter, Shigella, Entamoeba histolytica and Lymphogranuloma venereum and Chlamydia trachomatis. Gonorrhea generally involves the anus and <u>distal</u> rectum.

PITFALLS

1. Infectious proctitis in a homosexual male may be confused with ulcerative proctitis if a sexual history is not obtained. Such patients may be treated with corticosteroid enemas, an unfortunate choice for gonorrhea, herpes or other causes of the homosexual bowel.

2. Homosexual men who present with intestinal symptoms may have more than 1 pathogen.

3. Genital warts, found in 8-12% of homosexual men attending STD clinics, may have rectal as well as perianal involvement. There is a high recurrence rate after the usual therapy of podophyllin, cryotherapy or surgery.

SUGGESTED READINGS

Andrews H, Wyke J, Lane M, et al: Prevalence of sexually transmitted disease among male patients presenting with proctitis. Gut 29:332, 1988.
Burkes RL, Meyer PR, Gill PS, et al: Rectal lymphoma in homosexual men. Arch Int Med 146:913, 1986.
Daling JR, Weiss NS, Hislop TG, et al: Sexual practices, sexually transmitted diseases, and the incidence of anal cancer. N Engl J Med 317:973, 1987.
Laughon BE, Druckman DA, Vernon A, et al: Prevalance of enteric pathogens in homosexual men with and without acquired immunodeficiency syndrome. Gastroenterology 94:984, 1988.
Lebedeff DA, Hochman EB: Rectal gonorrhea in men: Diagnosis and treatment. Ann Int Med 92:463, 1980.
Weller IVD: The homosexual bowel. Gut 26:869, 1985.

Index